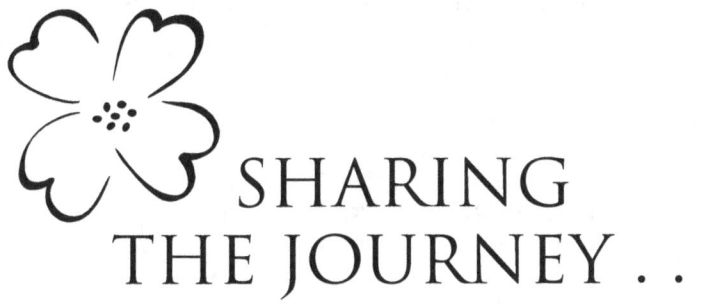

SHARING
THE JOURNEY . . .

The First Thirty Years of
Hospice of the Piedmont
1980–2010

R. TAL HAYNES

SHARING THE JOURNEY: THE FIRST 30 YEARS OF HOSPICE OF THE PIEDMONT, 1980–2010

By R. Tal Haynes

ISBN 978-1-4636499-2-0

Published by

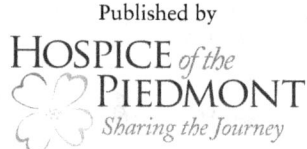

675 Peter Jefferson Parkway, Suite 300

Charlottesville, Virginia 22911

434.817.6900 • 800.975.5501

www.hopva.org

Editorial Production & Design: William Theodore Van Doren and Laura Owen Sutherland

TABLE OF CONTENTS

NAVIGATING THE AWKWARD SILENCE

George called, in panic mode. Someone in the college alumni office had talked him into taking over as our class secretary and his deadline for submitting bits of classmate news for the next edition of the alumni journal was only days away.

"Look, give me something. Anything. Like, what are you doing in retirement?"

"Retirement — what's that, George? I'm working full time in development and community relations for Hospice of the Piedmont in Charlottesville."

Awkward silence.

Finally, George mumbled, "So . . . how's your golf game coming along?"

When I was asked to compile a history of Hospice of the Piedmont for its thirtieth anniversary, I remembered that telephone call from my college classmate, and the awkward silence that followed my mention of hospice. I remembered, too, all the health fairs I had participated in over the years as we attempted to educate the public on the full scope of hospice care, and how so many of the attendees would look the other way as they walked by our display.

Those of us associated with hospice soon grow accustomed to the awkward silences and palpable discomfort hospice seems to elicit — a response engendered by a strange mixture of myth and fact in the public's understanding of hospice care. Even today, mention of hospice may do little more than serve as an unwelcome reminder of the big 'D'. I certainly suspect this may have been the case with my classmate, George. Indeed, for too many, still, hospice appears to be all about dying.

In reality, hospice is all about *living* — a holistic approach focused on empowering the patient and family, enhancing the physical, emotional and spiritual quality of the patient's life, and supporting the practical, emotional and spiritual needs of the entire family.

Admittedly, it was with some reluctance — or trepidation — that I accepted the challenge of creating this account of Hospice of the Piedmont's first thirty years. I knew it would be difficult to do justice to the extraordinary passion and commitment of its founders. In the face of tremendous obstacles, they refused over and over again to accept failure. Nor would it be a simple thing to convey the wonder of the compassionate care its staff has provided for more than 17,000 terminally ill patients and their loved ones since 1980 and the deep respect its commitment to excellence has earned throughout central Virginia and beyond. But for me the matter had been decided back in 1989, when my agreement to spend 12 weeks helping the struggling agency design a development program grew into a more than twenty-year tenure on its staff. I knew that the challenge of producing a book for the thirtieth anniversary of this exceptional agency's service in central Virginia was one I could not refuse.

Chapter 1

WHEN IT'S UP CLOSE AND PERSONAL

Six years into my work with Hospice of the Piedmont in Charlottesville, Virginia, I had learned a great deal about hospice care. However, most of it was "head knowledge." I had yet to experience the deeper "heart knowledge" that comes from personal encounter. I begin this history of Hospice of the Piedmont with a bit of my family history that transformed my understanding of the real wonder of hospice care.

My journey to real understanding began on a hot, muggy morning in July 1995. The head nurse at the assisted living facility had discovered a lump on my mother's breast. Within two weeks, a needle biopsy confirmed our worst fears — my 90-year-old mother had cancer.

As hospice director of development and public relations, I could recite the extraordinary care and services we provided chapter and verse, backwards and forward — it had become old hat. For the better part of six years, I had written about it, talked about it, designed fundraisers for it — I considered myself a true believer. But, as I was about to discover, believing something to be wonderful is one thing — seeing that wonder up close and personal can be quite another.

Speaking into her good ear, the oncologist told Mom she had breast cancer. Smiling pensively, she said, "Well, that's no good."

She always did have a penchant for understatement.

Giving her a gentle pat on the back, he recommended that she undergo a modified mastectomy. Often confused, Mom was clear as a bell on this. "Oh, I'm much too old for surgery." She was still smiling, but there was no doubt her decision was final.

The doctor chuckled and offered her a deal.

"Let's try some oral chemotherapy for a few weeks and see if it helps. If it doesn't, we'll talk some more about having it removed, O.K.?"

Mom smiled and nodded. With her hearing problem, she routinely smiled and nodded when spoken to and I wondered if she had really understood what he was saying.

Over the ensuing weeks, it became evident that the oral chemotherapy was not having the desired effect. The mass, close to the surface of the skin, was growing and had begun to drain. Pain control was becoming a problem and there were days when Mom was too weak to dress herself or go to meals. There was talk of transferring her to the nursing wing, but no beds were available. The options had run out and, after much discussion with Mom, the mastectomy was scheduled.

As part of the pre-op examination, the surgeon ordered a chest X-ray. To our dismay, it showed that the cancer had already spread to her lungs. It was obvious that the situation was hopeless and the operation was cancelled. By this time, Mom had forgotten the discussion about surgery and, within a few days, while remaining in her retirement facility, she became a hospice patient.

The first day after she was admitted as a patient, she was visited by a hospice social worker and a hospice nurse. It was noted that Mom was experiencing an increased level of breakthrough pain. By nightfall, the nurse had been in touch with the oncologist, who ordered a needed adjustment in Mom's pain control medication. On the second day, a hospice chaplain was there for a long visit and arrangements got underway for regular visits from a trained hospice volunteer. I watched as they took over Mom's physical, emotional and spiritual care with skill and compassion.

It is difficult to convey the profound sense of relief I experienced in knowing my mother was being cared for by these professionals committed to her comfort and well-being. Each of them also sought me out, explaining the plan of care their interdisciplinary team would be providing with the physician's approval and inquiring about any needs my wife and I might have as we dealt with her limited life expectancy.

Things took a sudden turn a short time later when Mom had a massive heart attack. By the time the retirement facility reached me that Saturday morning, Mom was being transported by ambulance to Martha Jefferson Hospital. Rushing into the emergency entrance of the hospital, I was directed to the cubicle where members of the emergency room staff were working to stabilize Mom. Barbara, my wife, had arrived a few minutes before and was holding Mom's hand.

When the medical team had done what it could to make Mom more comfortable, I let the physician in charge know that my mother was a hospice patient. She was taken up to the fifth floor and down a corridor where, at that time, Hospice of the Piedmont staffed a six-bed inpatient unit — "Hospice of the Piedmont at Martha Jefferson." The weekend hospice staff quickly took over her care.

After being moved from the gurney to the comfortable bed, she spotted the huge oak tree outside her window, its leaves resplendent with the brilliant hues of autumn. She smiled and, with a touch of awe in her voice, said, "What a beautiful tree!" That was the last thing I ever heard her say.

Working with her oncologist, the hospice staff saw to it that she remained pain free and, even after she had slipped into a coma, they continued to talk to her gently, aware that she might be hearing them. Shortly before noon the next day, Mom slipped away quietly and peacefully.

I was left with a new dimension in my understanding of hospice care. In spite of the comparatively brief time Mom was a patient of Hospice of the Piedmont, I came to know, in ways I could not otherwise have fathomed, the tremendous difference hospice can make to the quality of life of the patient and to the peace of mind of the entire family.

No, Hospice of the Piedmont did not cure my mother's cancer. As far as I know, it did not add five minutes to her life. But it did provide some things that were infinitely valuable and worthwhile: it enriched her last days, physically and spiritually, and, when the time came, it surrounded her with skilled, compassionate health care professionals who enabled her to die without the pain that had increasingly ruled her life before she became a hospice patient.

And there was something else — something I almost hesitate to mention. Medical costs had been eroding her small financial resources for some time. But, from the moment she became a patient of Hospice of the Piedmont, all medical costs related to her terminal illness were borne by hospice — completely! Her medications, the expensive dressings that had to be changed several times each day, the injections, the morphine drip — all of it was taken care of by hospice. It was the final blessing that, among so many others, hospice provided for Mom and for those of us who loved her.

Yes, believing something to be wonderful is one thing; experiencing that wonder up close and personal can be quite another. I was left with the realization that the words we had once used on all our brochures to characterize hospice care were truer than I had realized:

"There when the need is greatest . . . "

❀ Chapter 2
A HISTORICAL PERSPECTIVE

As far back as medieval times, the term "hospice" was used to indicate a place where weary or ailing travelers on a long journey could find shelter and rest. In 1967, Dame Cicely Saunders, then a young physician, applied the term to a concept of holistic care for terminally ill patients and their loved ones. She founded the first modern hospice, in a suburb of London — aptly naming it St. Christopher's Hospice, after the patron saint of travelers.

Cicely Saunders was a 21-year-old student at St. Anne's College, Oxford University, when World War II began in 1939. In 1940, she decided to suspend her studies to become a student nurse at St. Thomas Hospital in London. Soon, however, she suffered a back injury that eventually forced her to leave nursing; in 1944 she returned to Oxford to complete the requirements for her BA. Having accomplished that and unable to resume an active nursing career, Cicely made the life-changing decision to enter training as a "hospital almoner," or medical social worker. It was while serving in this role at a London hospital in 1948 that she met and cared for David Tasma, a Polish-Jewish refugee and survivor of the Warsaw ghetto.

Tasma was dying with cancer. Although they knew each other only a short time, a deep friendship developed — indeed, it is generally agreed that they fell in love. In any event, Cicely was inspired and energized by their long discussions about the need for a more holistic approach to caring for the terminally ill — addressing not only the medical concerns of those close to the end of life, but also their emotional and spiritual needs. They spent long hours discussing the sort of setting where this kind of care could best be provided — places more like home.

As the end of his short life approached, David Tasma presented Cicely Saunders with a gift of £500 (around $750) as the first donation toward building the kind of place they had envisioned. "Perhaps I can be a window in your Home," he said. He died February 25, 1948.

Determined to immerse herself in further study of the needs of terminally ill patients, Cicely Saunders volunteered to work at St. Luke's, a home for the dying in London. Over a period of time, she arrived at the conclusion that, in order to make the greatest impact on the culture of care for those at the end of life, she would have to become a physician. So it was that this determined nurse and medical social worker became a research fellow at St. Mary's School of Medicine. Working and conducting research at St. Joseph's Hospice in London's east end, she established the basic principles of modern hospice care, with its attention to innovative pain control and support of the social, emotional and spiritual needs of patients and their families — principles that would cause her to become recognized as the founder of modern hospice care and a major pioneer in the field of palliative medicine.

Finally, after a lengthy period of planning and fund-raising, the dream she and David Tasma had shared became a reality as St. Christopher's Hospice opened to receive its first patients in 1967. David Tasma's gift is commemorated by a plain sheet of glass in the entrance to the hospice. Reflecting on the long journey, Cicely Saunders said, "It took me 19 years to build the home round the window."

Two years after the opening of St. Christopher's, a book by Dr. Elisabeth Kübler-Ross, *On Death and Dying,* was published in the United States. Based on over 500 interviews with dying persons, the book became an internationally known best seller. In the book, Kübler-Ross made the case for the provision of home care as opposed to treatment in an institutional setting and argued that dying patients should have a choice and a voice in decisions affecting their destinies. Kübler-Ross would later testify at the first national hearings on death with dignity, conducted by the U. S. Senate Special Committee on Aging in 1974. She decried the practice of institutionalizing and isolating the old and dying in our "death-denying society" and spoke of the need for spiritual, emotional and financial help to make home care possible at the end of life.

Meanwhile, a chain of events had been set in motion that would result in bringing modern hospice care to the United States.

Florence Wald, dean of the Yale School of Nursing, invited Cicely Saunders to become a visiting faculty member for the spring term of 1965. She became intrigued by Dr. Saunders' concept of holistic hospice care and her use of palliative care for terminally ill cancer patients as a way of enabling them to focus on their personal relationships as they prepared for death. Saunders' practice of controlling pain in these patients by administering opioids "on the clock," rather than waiting until pain erupted, was a new concept.

Wald subsequently traveled to England several times, spending considerable time with Cicely Saunders and observing the innovative care provided at St. Christopher's. Back at Yale, she organized a team of doctors, clergy and nurses to study the needs of the dying and, in 1974, along with several doctors and a Yale medical center chaplain, founded the first hospice in America, the Connecticut Hospice, in Branford, with funding from the National Cancer Institute.

Four years later, as residents of Charlottesville and Albemarle County leafed through the October 1, 1978, edition of *The Daily Progress*, they would have come upon a full-page article by staff writer Sara Bullard on the distinguished career of Dr. Cicely Saunders and news of her forthcoming appearance at the University of Virginia on October 4th. No account of the history of Hospice of the Piedmont would be complete without reference to that whirlwind visit of Cicely Saunders and the seeds she sowed through the force of her personality and the passion of her commitment to change the culture of end-of-life care. Without question, the impetus for the founding of Hospice of the Piedmont grew out of that one-day visit in 1978.

After serving on an afternoon panel discussion on "Hospice Care: The Nature and Management of Terminal Illness," Cicely Saunders delivered The Zula Mae Bice Memorial Lecture at Fenwick Auditorium, McLeod Hall and, that evening, showed her film, *Hospice*, at St. Paul's Memorial Church on University Avenue. Then she was off to Washington, D.C., where she would speak the next morning at the first annual meeting of the National Hospice Organization, at the Shoreham Americana Hotel. Senator Edward M. Kennedy of Massachusetts was the keynote speaker at that meeting and, no doubt with a nod in the direction of Cicely Saunders, said this about the evolving hospice movement in the United States: "The hospice movement is a great movement, not because it was legislated by Congress, or mandated by the Federal Government, but because it evolved out of the hearts of people who care."

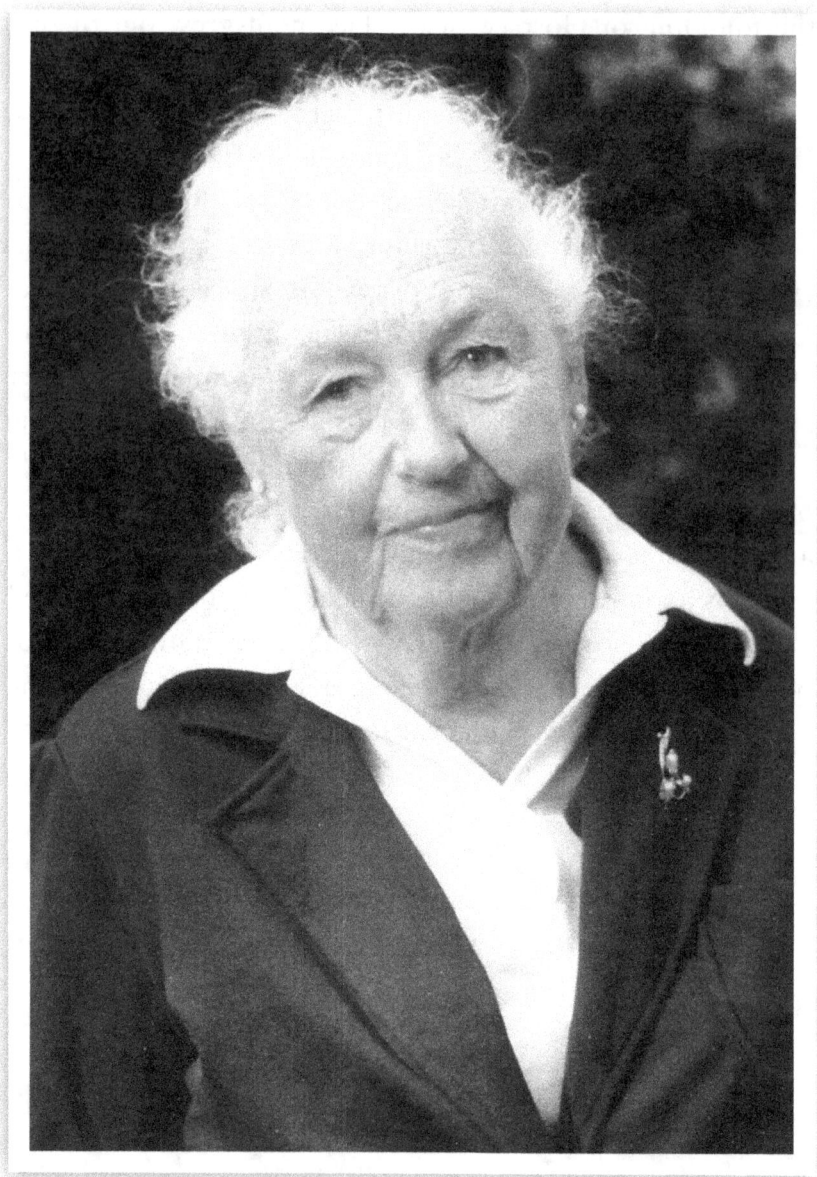

Adge Coburn.

$\mathbb{G}$ *Chapter 3*

INSPIRATION AND HARD WORK

I n the months following Cicely Saunders' 1978 visit, a group of persons intrigued by the hospice concept began meeting together in Charlottesville — often at the home of Agnes "Adge" Coburn. If the history of Hospice of the Piedmont could not be written without reference to the impact of Cicely Saunders' whirlwind visit, neither could it be compiled without acknowledging the pivotal role of Adge Coburn in its founding.

Born in Paterson, N.J., on May 30, 1910, Adge was a graduate of The Masters School in Dobbs Ferry, N.Y., and received her R.N. degree from Columbia Presbyterian School of Nursing. She and her husband, Alvin Frederick Coburn, MD, a noted rheumatologist whose last academic appointment was in the department of medicine at the University of Virginia, moved to Charlottesville in 1968.

Following the cancer-related death of her second daughter, Sarah Coburn, Adge became very interested in the hospice movement and began traveling widely, collecting information about hospice programs throughout the United States and Canada. Dr. George Cooper, who became the first president of Hospice of the Piedmont's board, was fond of calling Mrs. Coburn "The Instigator." Indeed, the group that, more often than not, gathered at her home outside of Charlottesville to discuss creating a hospice, owed much to her persistence. She was not about to let the dream die.

There is no written account of the activities of this group until May 28, 1980. On that evening, the group gathered at Mrs. Coburn's home. Thirty persons are listed as members of the group, twenty of whom were present that evening, with the stated purpose of "furthering the idea of a Hospice to care for the terminally ill patients and their families within the area known as Planning District #10."

Rosemary Hayes, RN, reported on a training program underway for thirteen volunteers who wished to become directly involved in the care program. Dr. George Cooper, a highly respected radiologist, reported on a conversation with John Harlan of the University of Virginia Hospital indicating that beds for hospice would probably not be available there. However, there was a group consensus that beds might well be made available at Martha Jefferson Hospital.

At that point, the meeting "turned to the business of authorizing a group of responsible officers to expedite the machinery of the organization." Dr. Cooper was unanimously elected president; Mrs. Adge Coburn, vice president; Mrs. Asha Greer, secretary; and Mrs. Pat Llewellyn, treasurer. There followed "considerable discussion as to the name of whatever organization emerges. Since no one wishes to limit our involvement within reasonable bounds, it was felt best to adopt something like 'Hospice of the Piedmont', pending the approval of the National Hospice Organization." This May 1980 meeting is described in subsequent minutes as "the original board meeting."

As the result of some conversations to which we are not privy, the newly elected vice president and secretary were granted the Board's permission to exchange offices — which explains why the official minutes of Hospice of the Piedmont's initial years were written by Adge Coburn. Her carefully written minutes and other correspondence are a treasure — sometimes overflowing with excitement and emotion, often filled with editorial remarks, sometimes cajoling the board and staff to keep on keeping on because what they were doing mattered so much, and, always, revealing her personal commitment and enthusiasm for establishing hospice care in central Virginia.

The following excerpts from a newsletter she composed and sent to the board in early September 1980 are typical. (Note that her mention of the "new Connecticut Hospice" refers specifically to the newly completed inpatient unit of America's first hospice, which had been founded in 1974.)

And now with a hot and humid summer more or less behind us, we hope, it is time for getting on with the job. You will all be interested in a brief summary of happenings during the last two months and it follows here:

My son and I, en route to Maine on June 29th, were near enough to the new Connecticut Hospice in Branford (near New Haven) to include it on its opening — Dedication Day. It is a very interesting building, in design extremely contemporary and functional. Furnishings and interior decoration were also modern. All beds are in units of four and are surrounded by large glass areas, i.e., on each wall and overhead. The patient rooms face undeveloped woodland with a modern Episcopal church in the distance. Much will be made of the use of plants, standing, hanging, on shelves, on the patios (outside of all patients' rooms and accessible to them) and in the landscaping not yet complete. Other facilities include a library, dining room, living rooms for each four-bed unit, chapel, music room, and, of course, kitchens, offices, scream room and 'viewing room'. The latter I could have done without. But they have really thought of everything.

On our own home front, Nancy Stamm (our legal advisor) has done a major job. She has masterminded our Articles of Incorporation and they are now under consideration by the State Corporation Commission. Hopefully they will be approved and then we can apply to the IRS for tax-exempt status. Then we shall be free to bring our efforts to the notice of the public and ask for help.

Out of the blue during August came a cordial note from Dr. Cowen Ellis, Pastor of the First Baptist

Church, offering to help in any way he could. I have met and talked with him in their beautiful new church. Dr. Ellis has agreed to serve on our Board.

Your Executive Committee has approved of my participation in the forthcoming Hospice Seminar in Montreal sponsored by the National Hospice Organization and the Royal Victoria Hospital from October 6–8. My purpose is to glean as much knowledge and information as I can and to pick up as many crumbs from the professionals as possible. It always helps to keep our problems and our faces before their eyes so that when we need them they will remember us. People involved in this movement, volunteers or professional are <u>always</u> ready to give the weaker member a helping hand. It is a very heartening experience. Pat Llewellyn and Sarah Hendley are planning to attend the annual meeting of the Virginia Association of Hospices to be held in Williamsburg on October 2–3 for the same reasons. We now belong to this group.

The volunteers who completed the first series of indoctrination lectures on hospice care agreed to continue meeting in order to attend Mrs. Palmer's course in Home Nursing. The course was held and those volunteers who attended felt that the experience was well worth it.

So you see, we just might 'get all our ducks in line' in the not too distant future, so be of good cheer and have faith because we are all working together.

THE FIRST THIRTY YEARS

Hospice of the Piedmont owes a tremendous debt to Adge Coburn and that small founding group who shared her passion for providing hospice care for the terminally ill of central Virginia.

By the spring of 1981, it had become evident that a full-time executive director and a patient coordinator would soon be needed. Area interest was running high and a growing number of invitations to speak to community groups on the concept of hospice care were being received, as well as a number of requests for patient care. The board was continuing to focus its attention on basic organizational tasks such as the crucial issue of securing adequate insurance coverage for board members and volunteers, exploring the possibilities for assistance from existing community organizations, such as the Public Health Department and the American Red Cross, and finding permanent office space.

Chapter 4

A DAY TO REMEMBER

At noon on April 15, 1981, Dr. George Cooper called the board meeting to order in the conference room of the Thomas Jefferson Health Department. The meeting would be a historic one, where all the months of effort began to bear fruit. These excerpts from Adge Coburn's minutes reflect an unbridled sense of joy:

Your kindly understanding of these minutes is requested by your secretary who is so euphoric over the momentous impact of the decisions arrived at therein that she is having great difficulty reporting the facts. So be it.

1. Our request for tax-exemption to the IRS has been granted as of April 14. Now we may request funds with a clear conscience.

2. A fund-raising committee headed by Carr Dorman [subsequently changed to Buck Carnan] has been suggested and approved. This committee has been instructed by the president to raise sufficient funds to enable us to employ an executive director for several months, one of whose functions will be to launch a major fund-raising drive in order to give us a secure base of operations. Therefore, it is understood that this first effort at fund raising will be low profile, no major publicity, person-to-person solicitation. It is expected that the board members will each contribute.

3. The Chairman discussed the main points of Miss Jane Alan's proposal from the American Red Cross to assist in the launching of hospice. However, since the points mentioned above and the points following obviate the need for our involvement with another service agency, it was understood that we no longer needed their assistance. A letter thanking the American Red Cross for their cooperation will be sent, and it is hoped that our friendly cooperation will continue.

4. The question of insurance was brought up by Jack Darrell, who had invited Bruce Cabell to be present in order to address this matter. He presented a proposal which would provide general liability coverage for injury to persons and/or property. This would protect the association, Board members and volunteers for an annual cost of $300. A smaller commitment of $50 covering automobile liability was also accepted.

5. Dr. Gleason reported that the Martha Jefferson Hospital board was much in favor of implementing the hospice concept of care. He believes they will commit some beds for hospice use in the near future. It seems that there is a possibility that Blue Cross may choose to support this effort as a pilot study. Dr. Cooper was authorized to speak to the MJH board on our behalf at their next meeting.

6. We were asked to decide whether we were now ready to accept patients for the present and that an evaluation of their care be made at the end of two months. Dr. Cooper instructed the patient care coordinators to work together with the Public Health Department and, to that end, signed an Agreement between Hospice and the Health Department that had been drawn up by Mrs. Mary McGee.

7. The four instructors of volunteers present as guests (Joy Spalding, Nina Todor, Sherri McCabe, John Ashley) were then introduced and were warmly thanked for their help with the volunteers. Also present as guests were Ann Bunts (P.H. Nurse) and Dela Alexander.

A box lunch was provided by members of the board. The meeting adjourned at 1:00 P.M.

Shortly after this meeting, Hospice of the Piedmont began to provide care for its first two patients, both with cancer — a middle-aged father of eight and a 50-year-old mother of a school-age child. The volunteer's notes on Mr. "M" refer to this case as a success "in that the team worked itself out of a job. Our prompt, caring attention gave moral support, which is all we could discover the family needed . . . . the children recovered from shock and rallied, understanding that their presence is the comfort their parents need . . . . We are no longer strangers; if they panic again, they will feel free to call us. I will stay in touch with the family without invading their privacy."

Following Mr. "M's" death, bereavement counseling got underway for this large family.

The case of the mother with a school-age child is moving. She was thought to have only a few months to live and was receiving 16–18 hours of volunteer services weekly, in addition to Public Health nurse visits. Her volunteer's notes indicate that one of the patient's primary concerns was for her 10-year-old daughter. She lived for eighteen months — not ready to die until she could feel at peace about her ten-year-old daughter, who was to be raised by her grown son and his wife.

Sarah Hendley, MSW, who was helping to train and to coordinate volunteer services at the time, wrote: "Several nurses at Martha Jefferson Hospital called to tell me that her dying was the most peaceful they had ever witnessed, thanks to the loving care of Mag (Margaret) Robinson and Joan Barnochy, who supported the patient and her family as hospice volunteers at home and in the hospital."

And so, after all the months of preparation, it began — with loving, compassionate attention to the special needs of two terminally ill patients and their loved ones. Many things would change in the years ahead, but not the essence of hospice care as seen in these early volunteers. Truly, then as now, volunteers have been "the heart" of hospice.

A NEW ERA

Two milestones were reached during 1981 that signaled a
new era in the development of Hospice of the Piedmont
— the leasing of a professional office space and the hiring, at
long last, of the first executive director.

The original hospice "office" is described by an early
volunteer as "a small space for a desk and phone within a large
basement meeting room of the then Senior Center, located in
the red brick insurance building at 101 High Street." When
the Senior Center announced it would be moving into the
old McIntire Library building in June, 1981, hospice began a
search for a more permanent space. The search led to a new
home in two offices on the second floor of Chauncey Hutter's
Tax Service building at 205 2nd Street, S.W., near what is
currently the Mono Loco Restaurant.

By far the most important milestone reached in 1981 was the
arrival of the new executive director, the Reverend Dinah Ansley,
on October 1, 1981. Dinah had previously served as executive
director of United Cerebral Palsy in Jacksonville, Florida and,
closer to home, as executive director of the newly established
Jefferson Area Board for Aging (JABA) in Charlottesville.

While in graduate school at Yale, Dinah had worked as a planner/programmer for New Haven's Elderly Services and earned a Master's in rehabilitative counseling with a minor in administration and supervision. More recently, Dinah had earned a second Master's degree, from Yale Divinity School. It was while at Yale that she had classes with the director of the Hospice of Connecticut and became very familiar with and excited about the hospice concept. Prior to becoming Hospice of the Piedmont's first executive director, she had been ordained by Blue Ridge Presbytery and was serving as minister of the Rustburg Presbyterian Church.

Dinah Ansley assumed the position of executive director at a very pivotal time in the history of hospice care in America. Congress included a provision to create a Medicare hospice benefit in the Tax Equity and Fiscal Responsibility Act of 1982, with a 1986 sunset provision. Congress made the benefit permanent in 1986, gave states the option of including hospice in their Medicaid programs, and made hospice care available to terminally ill nursing home residents.

The board was initially reluctant to seek certification by the Health Care Financing Administration (HCFA) to offer the Hospice Medicare benefit to eligible patients and their families. It was feared that involvement with governmental bureaucracy would result in a great deal of unnecessary red tape and could, over time, have a negative effect on the autonomy of local hospice programs. It would not be until the spring of 1988 that the Board of Directors would vote to seek certification to offer care under the Hospice Medicare Benefit.

Shortly after the arrival of Dinah Ansley, the hospice office moved from its two-room office on 2nd Street, S.W. into a five-room house at 908 Sycamore Street. The house, owned by Martha Jefferson Hospital, was rented to Hospice of the Piedmont for the princely sum of $1.00 a year.

At the March 1983 annual meeting, retiring board president George Cooper, MD, was honored for his service and guidance to Hospice of the Piedmont. William R. Sandusky, MD, retired professor of surgery, was welcomed as his successor.

Dinah Ansley's tenure as executive director extended from 1981 to the early spring of 1985 — a time with its share of financial concerns and fears that the whole endeavor could fail. The Fall 1983 newsletter begins with these words: "Hospice of the Piedmont is on the brink of extinction unless overwhelming financial support is forthcoming from individuals, churches, foundations and social organizations." But, as has been the case so often in the history of Hospice of the Piedmont, this desperate need was met with unbelievable generosity — some $40,000 in individual gifts, an anonymous challenge gift of $25,000 for endowment, and a matching $25,000 from the W. Alton Jones Foundation.

Dinah Ansley's tenure was marked by courage, determination and a refusal on the part of the board and staff to accept failure. What are her impressions of those years?

"I remember Adge Coburn and her passion as she carted me around the state looking at the few hospice programs that were just beginning in Virginia. I remember her fortitude as she organized, spoke on behalf of, and even arm-twisted when necessary for the development and long life of Hospice of the Piedmont.

"I remember volunteers — volunteers who served for years, aiding families and patients during snowstorms and blistering heat and holidays and ordinary days — with such compassion, such commitment, such generosity of heart.

"I remember Carol Jones — the first official 'Volunteer Coordinator', who labored endlessly doing all kinds of things she really didn't like, but was so loyal to hospice, to the volunteers, and to the patients and family members.

"I remember someone dying — and the energy in the room becoming absolutely transformed — and my mind opening to the possibility of other dimensions of reality that we do not readily see.

"I remember the Board of Directors — sincere, earnest, enthusiastic, faithful, trusting . . . .

"I remember the first piece of correspondence I received as executive director — addressed to "The Hot Spice of the Piedmont," and the countless talks I gave educating the public about hospice care and hospice philosophy.

"I remember bleakness and no money and the fear of having to close Hospice — and the appearance of two angels: first Laura West — a nurse who was willing to work for next to nothing (in fact, nothing to begin with) and be on call 24/7, and with gentleness and compassion and wisdom, guide folks on their final journey. And almost simultaneously, Karen Horridge, who picked up the reins as volunteer coordinator and a thousand other tasks that had no job description.

"I remember learning how someone working with patients needed to know physical care skills — and took a course to earn certification as a nursing assistant.

"I remember the first Virginia Association for Hospices conference with several hundred persons pre-registered — and Elisabeth Kübler-Ross's farm manager calling me the night before Elisabeth was to give the keynote address. He told me that she might not be able to make it because the ewes were lambing. I remember 30 minutes before the keynote address was to be delivered, this small, slightly stooped woman dressed in dirty jeans and muddy boots made her way into the conference center and, on cue, walked up to the podium and wowed the audience.

"And, what I continue to remember almost daily is my gratitude for the privilege of serving as the founding executive director of Hospice of the Piedmont and the pride I experience when I hear about its work and service now."

Following her resignation in the spring of 1985, Dinah returned to the pulpit, serving as minister of the Rockfish Presbyterian Church. She began to see the need for homecare in the Rockfish Valley and, easing out of the pulpit, began tending critically and terminally ill people in their homes and using her skills on the Appalachian dulcimer and banjo playing music for and with them. Simultaneously, she served as Artist-in-Residence at the UVa Cancer Center, providing music and comradeship for those who came there for treatment. Currently, she is on call for transporting friends and neighbors to radiation and chemotherapy treatments and organizes musical programs in Waynesboro, Virginia.

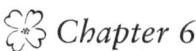 *Chapter 6*

THE HOSPICE ANGELS

It would be easy to believe that Brett Harrell was predestined to move across country and become Hospice of the Piedmont's second executive director. One could even imagine that the personal obstacles and trials he faced once he got to Charlottesville were somehow designed as a sort of training to temper his patience and determination for the challenges he would face in his new role.

Brett was comfortably situated as executive assistant to the president of the College of Idaho in 1983 when his wife, Sheila, received word that she had been accepted in a doctoral program in psychology at the University of Virginia. Assuming he would have no difficulty finding a job in another college community, Brett resigned his position at College of Idaho and he and Sheila set out for Charlottesville, arriving in time for the beginning of her studies in the early fall of 1983.

After months of fruitless searching, Brett had still found no suitable job opening; reluctantly, he and Sheila concluded that he should temporarily return to the College of Idaho, where his previous position was being held open for him. Over the next nine months, he balanced his work in Idaho with periodic flights back to Charlottesville to continue his job search. Finally, Sheila saw a classified advertisement for an executive director for Hospice of the Piedmont. She hurried to the telephone to call Brett.

As it happened, Brett had become extremely interested in the hospice concept because of his grandmother's terminal illness, which had led him to read everything he could find on hospice care. In the early months of his job search in Charlottesville, he had made a point of visiting the hospice office on Sycamore Street and meeting the members of its small staff. Instinctively, Sheila sensed this opening at Hospice of the Piedmont might signal the end of Brett's long search.

Brett immediately called the hospice office and spoke with one of the staff members he had met. The search for an executive director was just beginning, and Brett was encouraged to contact the search committee. In short order, Brett had applied for the position and was invited to fly to Charlottesville for an interview.

Brett chuckles as he recalls the day of his interview with Hospice of the Piedmont's large 30-member Board of Directors. Dinah Ansley escorted Brett from the Hospice office to Martha Jefferson Hospital, where two small meeting rooms had been reserved that day for the board's use. Brett wondered why the board, even as large as it was, would need two rooms for the interview, until he was introduced to a young man who, as it turned out, was also to be interviewed!

As Brett describes it, the scene was hilarious — he and the other candidate sat in a waiting area until directed to separate meeting rooms to be interviewed. Greeting each other as they returned to the waiting area, they chatted to pass the time until they were each ushered into the alternate meeting rooms.

Later that day, Brett met with the entire Board. When asked why he was interested in hospice, he spoke at length about his grandmother's illness and how she was dying in a little county hospital in east Tennessee and how she was simply terrified. He told them how he had read everything he could find on the hospice philosophy and the satisfaction he would receive from helping to make this special kind of care available for people like his grandmother.

The Board voted that very afternoon to hire him.

Brett's sense of humor was legendary. He seldom missed an opportunity to tell people that his first day on the job as executive director in 1985 was April Fools Day. After a suitable pause, he would say that he suspected that this was not merely a coincidence when he discovered that there was just enough money in the bank to pay the four-person staff for two more months!

"But," he would add, "I soon found out that there are special angels who watch over hospice — that's their full time job!"

That belief may date back to the early weeks of Brett's service as executive director when he heard about a lady who had just moved to Charlottesville and was asking around about local charity needs. Reaching her by telephone, Brett introduced himself and made an appointment to come to her home and discuss the needs of Hospice of the Piedmont.

He had a delightful visit and, within a few days, received a letter affirming her support of hospice and her personal check for $25,000.

Special angels, indeed!

As Brett settled into his position in 1985, Edmund "Ned" Morris was elected to succeed William Sandusky as president of the board. When Ned found it necessary to resign that position in 1986, John R. Metz, director of pharmacy services at Martha Jefferson Hospital, was elected to fill his unexpired three-year term.

In response to the growing need for hospice services, the daily patient census grew significantly during 1985 and 1986 and, as professional staff were added to accommodate this growth, it became obvious that the small four-room house on Sycamore Street had been outgrown. Already, file cabinets were filling the closets and walkers and wheelchairs for loan to patients were filling every nook and cranny. In late 1986, a search got underway for more adequate administrative space. With Martha Jefferson Hospital's recent provision of rooms for those hospice patients who needed to be hospitalized, it was hoped that a larger property close to Martha Jefferson Hospital might be found for the staff. However, after months of searching the area near the hospital, no properties of the needed size and zoning, and reasonable price, had been found.

Then, in March 1987, Brett received word from the heirs of a former Hospice of the Piedmont patient that they were about to put her East Jefferson Street house on the market and wanted him to be aware of it beforehand. The letter indicated a special

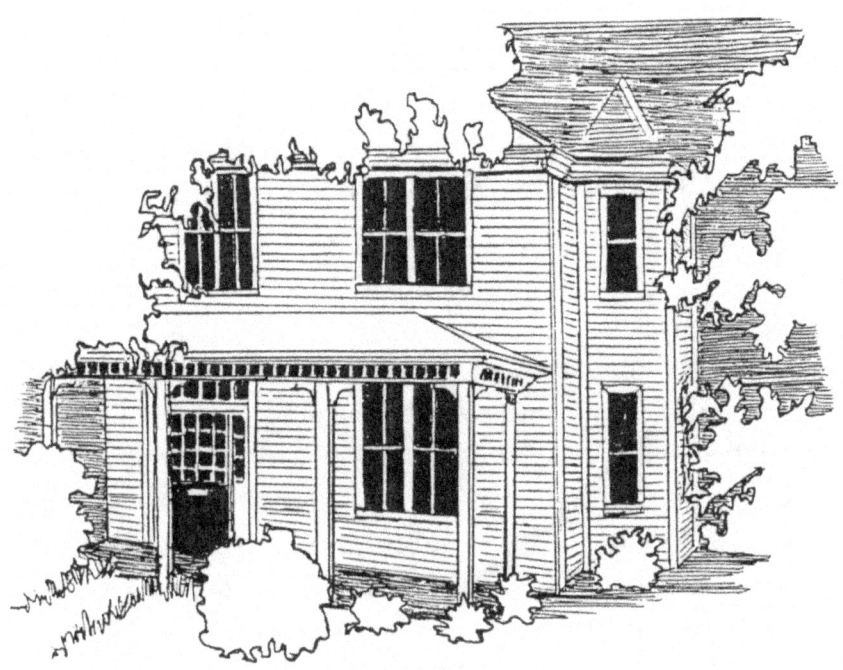

The house on East Jefferson Street.

bond the family felt with Hospice of the Piedmont because of the care given to their loved one in the house, including the presence of a hospice nurse when the patient had died there several years before. The Board quickly offered to purchase the 1925 Victorian-style house if funding could be found by the end of May. Shortly before the deadline, another "hospice angel" appeared — a local foundation agreed, anonymously, to provide the funds to purchase the house, with the understanding that Hospice of the Piedmont would be responsible for raising the funds necessary for renovation. The successful $75,000 fundraising and renovation took place over the next eight months and, in the last week of January, 1988, the staff moved into its new offices at 1002 East Jefferson Street, at the corner of 10th and Jefferson. It was to be a busy and pivotal year for Hospice of the Piedmont. Susan Garrett succeeded John Metz as president of the board and significant decisions would be made affecting the future growth and stability of hospice care in central Virginia.

Shortly after moving into its East Jefferson Street headquarters, the board — still reluctantly — began serious consideration of Medicare certification. Most of the original nucleus of founders resisted the move, fearing that any involvement with government bureaucracy would infringe on the heart of hospice. Brett Harrell, on the contrary, argued that the "heart of hospice" was exemplified by the quality of the people who worked and volunteered, not by the origin of funding. He was quick to say that he had not come to his support of Medicare certification easily, but had been driven to it by the growth in demand for hospice care and the corresponding need for increased funding to meet that demand in the future. As discussions continued, the board faced the fact that they were confronted with two options — either limit the number of patients or find new funding streams to allow staff and services to grow to meet the need. Finally, in June 1988, the board voted to seek Medicare certification.

If it were successful in becoming Medicare certified, Hospice would be compensated on a per diem basis for its care of eligible Medicare patients, while the Medicare Hospice Benefit would provide those patients with coverage that was unavailable from other parts of the Medicare program. This coverage would include, at no cost to the patient or family, all drugs related to the terminal illness, all equipment and supplies needed to keep the patient at home, and hospitalization for pain and symptom control if inpatient care became necessary. The hospice interdisciplinary team, composed of the family doctor, hospice nurses and social workers, volunteers, pastoral counselors, and other therapists as needed, would help the patient and family make decisions aimed at improving the quality of the life that remained to the patient, with the goal of allowing the patient to remain at home as long as possible.

In preparation for becoming Medicare certified, Brett contacted a number of certified hospices around the country, "stealing what I could from them to help in writing a policy and procedure manual." As he described it, "Sheila was in one room writing her dissertation and I was in another writing a policy and procedure manual for Medicare certification. I got that done in about four months and sent it in."

In late October, there was a two-day site visit by a Medicare official. Brett surmised that Medicare must have chosen the most difficult and demanding person on their staff to make the visit. The visit began with the announcement that she had locked the keys in her automobile and needed a locksmith. The two-day interrogation left Brett and the director of nursing, Ginny Kelly, totally exhausted — and, without a clue whether or not certification would be granted, they had to sit around and hold their breaths in the knowledge that the decision rested on this one official's shoulders.

Happily, word was received in December 1988 that Medicare provider status had been granted by the Health Care Financing Administration (HCFA). Hospice of the Piedmont, as an independent community-based hospice program, had become the first Medicare-certified hospice of its kind in the Commonwealth of Virginia.

In the spring of 1990, Brett Harrell submitted his resignation as executive director. He and Sheila were returning to Boise where she would begin to establish her counseling practice. Brett looked back on Medicare certification as the culmination of his tenure. "Financially, and in terms of building a foundation for everything else to sit on, the certification turned the whole operation around, providing enough income to begin expanding staff. I think of my five years there as a time of getting some of that initial foundation put in place and then, as my university president boss used to say, 'Brett, you want to be slipping quietly out the back door while the applause is still wafting in the wind.' "

As he and Sheila prepared to leave Charlottesville and return to Boise, Brett wrote his farewell article for the Spring 1990 issue of the newsletter *Hospice Happenings*. In it, he left this overview of his productive tenure as executive director and a glimpse of his warm and generous spirit:

"When I became Hospice of the Piedmont's second executive director in April 1985, we provided services that month to 19 families with one nurse and a part-time volunteer coordinator. Our offices were located in a tiny two-bedroom house on Sycamore Street owned by Martha Jefferson Hospital and leased generously to Hospice for $1.00 a year. We had enough money to meet two more monthly payrolls for our four-person paid staff. Some 70 hospice-trained volunteers were the foundation upon which our entire program rested — indeed, the only way it could operate.

"The caring group of people who are Hospice volunteers is about the only thing that hasn't changed in the past five years, except to become, thankfully, larger.

"This past April, we provided hospice care to 38 families, with more than half of them receiving the comprehensive services made possible by the Hospice Medicare Benefit. Our 12-person professional staff works out of our beautifully restored Victorian house on Jefferson Street, in which team meetings and support groups can comfortably be held. The UVa Medical Center has designated four beds in the new hospital for hospice patients, and other growing hospice programs from around Virginia contact us regularly seeking advice and assistance.

"Entering its second decade of service to central Virginia, Hospice of the Piedmont's future never looked brighter. It has been my privilege to have been a part of Hospice during a period of exciting growth and change, and to have worked closely with the many people who have contributed in their unique ways to keeping Hospice strong and stable throughout challenging and sometimes difficult times. My thanks to all who have made my journey with them so intensely rewarding, and my work with Hospice of the Piedmont the most fulfilling and joyful of my life."

One could never leave Brett's presence without receiving a smile and hearing him say, "Be careful." Perhaps it's because of that habitual admonition that his friends found the events of his departure from Charlottesville so amusing. On the day he and Sheila were to leave, Brett drove their fully loaded rental truck up to what was then the Central Fidelity Bank at Angus Road, planning to cash his final check from Hospice and get on the road to Boise. Pulling into one of the outdoor lanes at the bank, Brett carefully placed the check and his driver's license in the plastic cylinder and sent it up the vacuum tube to the teller across the way. He waited and waited until, finally, the teller's voice came on, asking if he could help him in any way.

"Well, yes," said Brett. "I'm waiting for my check to be cashed." Slowly, it dawned on the teller that whatever Brett had dispatched to him was stuck somewhere in the overhead vacuum tube. It was several hours later before a service crew arrived from Richmond to rescue the cylinder and its contents. Without question, the last thing the teller heard before the rental truck finally drove away was Brett's smiling admonition — "Be careful."

After his return to Boise, Brett became the state director of the Diabetes Association. He was later recruited by the State of Idaho to manage programs for newborn screening and special needs children. Now retired, Brett has a ready answer when asked what he is doing in retirement. With typical humor, he says, "Oh, I don't do much of anything, and some days, I don't get finished!"

❦ Chapter 7
GROWING UP FAST

Following Brett Harrell's resignation as executive director in May 1990, the Board of Directors moved quickly to elect staff member Ginny Kelly, RN, to succeed him. The director of nursing since 1988, Ginny had provided significant support to Brett in the process of seeking and implementing Medicare certification — and the board felt her to be an ideal choice as his successor.

A native of Long Island, Ginny received her Bachelor's of Science in nursing at Fairfield University in Connecticut and a dual Master's degree in public health and community health nursing from Boston University. Before moving to the Charlottesville area, she had worked as a pediatric nurse at Tuft's New England Medical Center in Boston and with Boston's Visiting Nurse Association in both staff and supervisory positions.

In her new role as executive director, Ginny would be working closely with a Board of Directors chaired by Gerald "Jerry" Bailey (1990–1992) and Richard A. Dershimer (1992–1995). One of Ginny's first hires was Patsy Tuffy, R.N., to fill the director of nursing position she had vacated.

A recent transplant to Charlottesville, Patsy had experience as both a field nurse and nursing director for home health nursing agencies in Philadelphia and Miami. Some years later, Patsy would become the executive director of Hospice of the Rapidan in Culpeper, Virginia.

With her staff of 12 and an average daily patient census of 35, Ginny and Hospice of the Piedmont embarked on a period of extraordinary growth and change. Looking back on her two years as director of nursing and three years as executive director, Ginny likens the early years of Hospice of the Piedmont to the development of a child.

"When Brett arrived, we were still in our infant stage — weak and wobbly. With his leadership, climaxed by our Medicare certification, we were beginning to be able to stand on our own two feet and take some tentative steps. By the time I became executive director, we had entered the toddler stage.

"Here," Ginny admits, "the analogy begins to break down. Hospice of the Piedmont did not remain a toddler for long and, rather than a slow, gradual blooming, it seemed to suddenly explode into adulthood. I became executive director at a very good time, when a lot of resources came together. Dr. John Lanham was established as a very active and popular medical director, Medicare certification was enabling us to hire a full complement of nurses and social workers and support staff and we had a great group of trained volunteers. Hospice seemed like a magnet in its ability to attract people who were intelligent, competent and caring — including board members, volunteers and staff. I feel very privileged to have served at the time when it was moving so rapidly into adulthood."

Indeed, even a cursory look at the events of her three-year tenure provides a sense of how rapidly events began to move. Soon after being named executive director, Ginny Kelly and her staff were involved in a lengthy survey process to become a licensed hospice program in Virginia. All Medicare-certified hospice programs in the Commonwealth were mandated to undergo this licensure process — one of the major benefits being the expansion of hospice services to recipients of Medicaid, the state-sponsored medical assistance program that is based on financial need. Hospice of the Piedmont successfully completed the process in August 1990, becoming one of the first licensed hospice programs in the state. The new Medicaid Hospice Benefit very closely mirrored the Hospice Medicare Benefit, providing for all medications, equipment, supplies and hospitalizations related to the person's terminal illness.

In addition, after nearly 10 years of negotiations, Blue Cross/Blue Shield signed a contract to include hospice patient services in their coverage. "Already," Ginny recalls, "with Medicare, Medicaid and Blue Cross/Blue Shield coverage, and the growing reputation of our 'special kind of caring', we were experiencing an increase in the number of families we were serving."

By the end of 1990, the staff of nurses, social workers and home health aides had driven 30,324 miles in providing over 4,500 hours of patient care; volunteers had documented another 21,261 miles and 3,421 hours of patient care.

As the staff grew to accommodate the growing demand for hospice care, there was a critical need for more office space. In October 1990, the Perry Foundation offered a $50,000 challenge grant for the construction of additional offices and an all-purpose meeting room on the second floor of the East Jefferson Street property. With the support of over 600 friends of Hospice, the $50,000 challenge grant was matched, the plans finalized, and the construction contract awarded to Abrahamse & Company Builders in December 1991. The new addition was completed in April 1992 and, by vote of the Board of Directors, was dedicated in loving memory of Adge Coburn, 81, who, sadly, had died on August 20, 1991, after a brief illness.

Ginny paid tribute to Adge in the Fall 1991 *Hospice Happenings*:

"Hospice of the Piedmont suffered a great loss in August when Agnes 'Adge' Coburn died. Those of us who were privileged to know firsthand of her deep devotion to hospice care will continue to be grateful for the many contributions she made to Hospice of the Piedmont. Gentle and self-effacing, Adge gave of herself generously, and never failed to take advantage of opportunities to promote hospice care in this community and beyond. Our debt to her is enormous. . . . Adge's efforts on behalf of Hospice of the Piedmont continued as the organization grew to meet the needs of our community. . . . As an active member of the Board of Directors, she played a significant role in the Board's mission of providing high-quality care for Charlottesville and the five-county area of Virginia Planning District Ten. She lived to see nearly 1,200 patients and families benefit from the 'special kind of caring' that sets hospice care apart in our society."

1992 was a year of tremendous growth and change for Hospice of the Piedmont. During that year, Hospice entered into contracts with two nursing homes to provide collaborative care to terminally ill patients and their families — an outreach that would include many additional nursing homes in the future. The building expansion, completed early in 1992, was expected to provide ample space for some time to come. However, by year's end, the daily patient census was nearing 60, the staff had doubled in size, and the enlarged office space was nearing full capacity.

As she looked ahead to the coming year, Ginny exhibited the can-do spirit that had been a part of the Hospice of the Piedmont psyche from the beginning.

"Although we have no way of knowing what changes 1993 may bring," she wrote, "we are certain that there are exciting and challenging days ahead. . . . Through it all, our commitment to provide the very highest level of care for our patients and their families will remain constant. . . . I take great personal encouragement from the competence and devotion of our staff and the outstanding leadership of our Board of Directors. Because of them, and the generous support of our many friends, I am confident we will be able to meet all the new challenges of the months ahead."

On Wednesday evening December 9, 1992, the first Hospice Tree ceremony was held on the grounds of the Charlottesville Omni Hotel with board president Dick Dershimer officiating. Hospice board and staff members joined families of hospice patients past and present along with community friends of hospice in this "Celebration of Life," as a large 15-foot evergreen tree, strung with hundreds of clear white bulbs, was lighted on the hotel grounds in memory and in honor of loved ones.

In the spring of 1993, Ginny Kelly announced that she and her husband were hoping to start a family soon and she would be leaving Hospice of the Piedmont in July. In her letter of resignation, she wrote:

"My five years of involvement with Hospice of the Piedmont have been challenging and rewarding. The growth and change I have been privileged to witness have been nothing less than remarkable. . . . I am convinced that Hospice of the Piedmont has thrived because of several interrelated factors: First of all, it has had the good fortune of attracting a staff of exceptionally compassionate, talented and dedicated persons. It has also had the guidance and support of outstanding community leaders serving on the Board of Directors. Added to that, a growing number of trained and devoted volunteers have shared their time and gifts to those in need. Finally, there has been a wonderful outpouring of support from all over our more than 2,000 square mile area of service. . . . With such devotion, the future of Hospice as a strong, effective organization is assured."

"Explosion" is perhaps as good a word as any for characterizing the growth and change that occurred during Ginny Kelly's three-year tenure as executive director. She began with a paid staff of 12, an average daily patient census of 35 and 146 patients cared for during the previous year. Three years later, the paid staff exceeded 40, the average daily census topped 80, and the number of patients cared for during the year was 288.

Today, Ginny continues with her nursing career, working part-time for a home health agency. She and her husband, John Moran, live in North Garden, Virginia, with their two teenaged sons, Austin and Will.

Chapter 8

TURBULENT TIMES

With Ginny Kelly's resignation, the Board asked Director of Nurses Patsy Tuffy to serve as interim executive director until a new executive director was in place. In light of the administrative and clinical challenges presented by the continued growth in the number of patients and patient families being served by Hospice of the Piedmont, the Board decided that a national search should be undertaken for a new executive director and stipulated that a masters degree in nursing, social work or business administration was preferred.

Board president Dick Dershimer was chosen to head up the search committee and was authorized to choose others to serve with him, including one member from the Hospice staff. The final committee membership included Jerry Bailey, Michael Bills, Pat Coffey, Betty Coyner, Susan Garrett, John Harlan, and staff member Jean Bradley, RN, the quality assurance nurse manager and supervisor of home health aides.

From a total of 41 applicants, the search committee recommended hiring Victoria Todd, MBA, executive director of the Naples, Florida, hospice, as Hospice of the Piedmont's new executive director. Vicky Todd was unanimously accepted and assumed her new position on August 30, 1993.

Vicky Todd became Hospice of the Piedmont's fourth executive director at a time of significant growth in the number of patients receiving hospice care in America and a rising recognition of the legitimate place of hospice in the nation's health care system. The number of hospices accredited to provide care under the Medicare Hospice Benefit had grown from 21 in 1984 to more than 1,288 in 1993 — some of the fastest growth occurring in home care agency–based and freestanding, community-based hospices like Hospice of the Piedmont. In that same year, hospice was proposed as a nationally guaranteed benefit under President Clinton's health care reform plan, reflecting the acceptance of hospice as part of the health care continuum. Nationally, a record 202,768 hospice patients received care under the Medicare Hospice Benefit in 1993. The following year, the Social Security Act Amendments required hospital discharge planners "to evaluate a patient's likely need for appropriate post-hospital services, including hospice services and the availability of those services."

All of this was very affirming for hospices in general, but some turbulent times lay just ahead for the hospice movement, and Hospice of the Piedmont would not be immune.

With the growing patient census, two geographical interdisciplinary teams were formed in late 1993 — one headed by Patient Family Care Coordinator Patsy Tuffy, the other by Jean Bradley. The average daily census was nearing

90 and the need for more office and meeting space had become an issue — three supervisors were sharing an office, there was no privacy for counseling staff or families, and no room for the additional liaison nurse, the second chaplain, and the finance director already being recruited.

The second annual Hospice Tree Celebration of Life was held December 1, 1993, on Charlottesville's downtown mall. Following a reception at Terry's Place, a restaurant just off the mall, hospice patient families, board members, staff, volunteers and friends of hospice made their way down to Central Place, where a large evergreen tree, strung with multi-colored bulbs, was lighted in memory or in honor of loved ones.

In February, 1994, negotiations were authorized for new office space. The staff was commended for its dedication and determination in meeting patient needs during that winter (1993–94), recognized as the harshest experienced in central Virginia in nearly two decades. It was noted that the staff made more than 1,000 visits to patients and families throughout Region 10 during the month of January alone.

Meanwhile, Vicky Todd was involved in ongoing negotiations with representatives of Martha Jefferson Hospital concerning development of a dedicated hospice unit managed by Hospice of the Piedmont within the hospital. In her March, 1994 report to the Board, she indicated that developing a financial arrangement that would be fair and acceptable to both entities was proving quite involved. She further reported that Fannie Utz, RN, had been hired as the second liaison nurse with primary responsibility at UVa Medical Center.

In late April, 1994, Dr. Marvin Barbre, an ordained minister and certified chaplain with extensive clinical pastoral training, became Hospice of the Piedmont's first full-time staff chaplain. With the patient census surging to 103 in early July, Barbara Lindsay, RN, became East Team leader, freeing Patsy Tuffy, RN, to provide overall nursing leadership for the program.

Several factors were contributing to the rapid growth in the number of patients, prime among them being an increase in nursing home referrals and the expanded area in which Hospice of the Piedmont was providing service. Initially, the service area had been confined to the City of Charlottesville and the five counties of Albemarle, Fluvanna, Greene, Louisa and Nelson. This was no longer true. By 1994, Hospice of the Piedmont was also caring for patients in Augusta and Buckingham counties, which at that time had no certified hospice programs, as well as for patients from the southern parts of Madison and Orange counties who were oriented to Charlottesville for medical care and who were referred by their physicians. Beyond these factors, perhaps more important in promoting its growth was the increasing awareness of Hospice of the Piedmont's unique role in the health care system, and its commitment to excellence of care.

In early summer, negotiations with Martha Jefferson Hospital were finalized and a contract signed, clearing the way for 'Hospice of the Piedmont at Martha Jefferson', a dedicated six-bed inpatient unit, to open August 1, 1994. For a number of years, hospice inpatient care had been provided at UVa Medical Center and Martha Jefferson Hospital through a "scattered bed" approach, i.e., hospice patients admitted to these facilities would be given whatever bed was available in the facility. With the opening of the dedicated inpatient unit, hospice patients at Martha Jefferson Hospital would all be in the special unit, redecorated for a homelike atmosphere and jointly staffed by Hospice and the hospital. Dr. Gordon Morris, an oncologist, agreed to serve as the unit's medical director, with Dr. John Lanham continuing as overall medical director of Hospice of the Piedmont.

Commenting on the new hospice unit, Vicky Todd said, "This new arrangement should improve continuity of care for hospice patients and provide a more peaceful refuge for their families. While dramatic, this change is but one example of our commitment to make certain that the patients and families we serve receive the best possible hospice care."

During 1994, HCFA sent out a memorandum alerting the nation's hospices to problems regarding questionable certifications and recertifications of terminal illnesses. This resulted in the first "focused medical review" for hospices and was a wake-up call to the industry to improve its documentation and certification procedures or be denied payments.

November 1, 1994 was moving day for Hospice of the Piedmont. Leaving its two-story Victorian home on East Jefferson Street, the burgeoning staff moved into a spacious office building on the corner of Westfield Road and Highway 29 North. At that month's board meeting, John Lah, the new director of finance, was introduced and approval was given for hiring a second full-time chaplain.

The board also received the sad news of the death of long-time volunteer and board member Margaret S. Robinson on November 4, 1994. A faithful volunteer since 1981, Maggie spent much of her 80 years helping others. In 1986, she was recognized by Hospice as Volunteer of the Year. In recent years, she had participated actively in the training of new volunteers and, at her death, was a member of the Board of Directors.

The third Hospice Tree Celebration of Life was held on the evening of December 6, 1994 at Fashion Square Mall. The ceremony featured the choir of St. Paul's Episcopal Church, Ivy, and the lighting of a 20-foot tree in memory and in honor of loved ones.

1995 was a very eventful year. By this time, the daily average of patients being cared for had leveled off at 130. Board member John F. Harlan, Jr., former executive director of UVa Hospital, succeeded Dick Dershimer as board president; Vicky Todd was authorized by the Executive Committee to engage in negotiations with UVa Hospital to establish a Hospice and Palliative Care unit; a second bereavement counselor position was approved to help staff member Beth Smith; and the second chaplain, the Reverend Karl Netting, began his work. The staff now totaled more than 100 full- and part-time employees and, to better deal with personnel issues, receptionist Pam Kimmel was named human resources specialist. Vicky commented, "Morale and productivity are quite high, but we do need to catch our collective breath and work on integrating all these new people into Hospice of the Piedmont in a meaningful way."

The Center for Hospice and Palliative Care at UVa was approved and slated to open in July 1995, with six rooms on 3 Central in the main hospital. Jane Griffith, RN, CRNH, an employee of Hospice of the Piedmont, was named the center's nurse administrator, with UVa's Carlos Gomez, MD, the medical director. The name of the center was chosen to highlight the strengths of both of the cooperating entities — hospice for its holistic approach to the physical, emotional and spiritual needs of terminally ill patients, as well as the practical, emotional and spiritual needs of their loved ones; UVa for its commitment to the emerging field of palliative medicine that focused on the treatment of pain and suffering as well as for the University's mission to teach and develop state-of-the-art medical knowledge and practices. Hospice chaplains would be working with their UVa counterparts to ensure that patients and their families received needed spiritual support, and trained Hospice volunteers would be on hand to visit and support patients and their families and assist staff. The establishment of the center represented a university/community relationship that was unique in the country at that time.

Typifying Hospice of the Piedmont's commitment to excellence in patient care, six Hospice RNs completed the requirements for special certification as Hospice Nurses during the summer of 1995: Karen Boyle, Jean Bradley, Anne M. Fromm, Jane Griffith, Sheila Johnson and Judy Smith. The prestigious Hospice Nurse certification (CRNH) is open to RNs only after two years of hospice service. After a great deal of study and preparation, done on their own time, the group traveled to Arlington, Virginia, to undergo a comprehensive four-hour examination that all of them passed with flying colors.

During the year, the Office of Inspector General (OIG) announced that Operation Restore Trust, a special program to combat waste and abuse in Medicare and Medicaid in five targeted states — California, Florida, Illinois, New York, and Texas — would be expanded to include hospice. Confident that the patient census would continue its steady growth, the Board adopted a budget for fiscal 1995–96 predicated on a patient census of 160. Soon thereafter, word was received of a 16% decrease in Medicare reimbursement, phased in over three years, beginning in October 1996.

The fourth Hospice Tree ceremony was held at Fashion Square Mall in early December, with board president John Harlan presiding. Once more, the choir of St. Paul's Episcopal Church, Ivy, participated in the program as a large 20-foot tree, donated by the mall and decorated by hospice volunteers, was lighted in memory and in honor of loved ones.

As a busy 1995 came to a close, Director of Nurses Patsy Tuffy, RN, tendered her resignation in order to accept her new position as executive director of Hospice of the Rapidan, headquartered in Culpeper, Virginia. Jane Griffith, RN, who had been with Hospice of the Piedmont since 1992, was named to succeed Patsy as director of nurses. Initially a liaison nurse, Jane had served as a bridge between Hospice, physicians, discharged planners and patients, and had played a significant role in the planning and opening of the inpatient unit at Martha Jefferson Hospital in August 1994. As noted, when the Hospice and Palliative Care Center opened at UVa Hospital a year later, Jane was appointed unit manager. Now this last appointment brought her back "in house" to assume the duties of the director of nurses, with Karen Boyle, RN, becoming the unit manager at UVa Hospital, and Dinah Pehrson-Day assuming the vacated liaison nurse position.

Medicare intermediaries on a national level were beginning to take a hard look at hospices and the large number of inpatient days billed under the Medicare Hospice Benefit. With beds now available at two comparatively new inpatient units, it is not surprising that Hospice of the Piedmont's inpatient admissions during fiscal 1995–96 showed a significant increase — catching the attention of the Medicare intermediary, who requested 30 patient charts for close review of the appropriateness of inpatient care.

At the same time, the intermediaries were focusing their attention on long-term patients with non-cancer diagnoses and, again, Hospice of the Piedmont's Medicare intermediary saw fit to pull a number of patient charts for review — a warning to hospice interdisciplinary teams to be more attentive to changes that might indicate a patient did not have, or no longer had, a hospice-appropriate prognosis of six months or less to live.

In the wake of the chart reviews and the directives coming out of HCFA and the OIG, referrals were declining and staff members, concerned about the future of Hospice of the Piedmont, were beginning to worry about their job security. The turbulence had begun.

In her report to the board on September 25, 1996, Vicky Todd expressed her concern over the amount of staff time and dollars devoted to the inpatient units during the past two years, and the change in focus the units had engendered: "We are seeing some patients for the first time when they enter the units — this is true of both units, but especially at UVa. Most of these patients never go home again."

To understand these concerns, one must remember that modern hospice care is provided by interdisciplinary teams of health care professionals with a goal of enabling patients to remain at home and of enhancing the quality of life by focusing on their physical, emotional and spiritual needs, as well as the practical, emotional and spiritual needs of their loved ones. This holistic approach requires a reasonable length of time to be fully effective for the patient and family — it takes time and trust to learn what dying patients and their families really want and need. The appropriate use of inpatient units, in this model, is for short-term symptom management, with the patient returning home after the symptom crisis has been brought under control. The units were not intended for brink-of-death care.

By the time Vicky Todd made this report to the board, the percentage of Hospice of the Piedmont's patients dying at home had decreased by 25%, and, more than any issue of staff time and dollars committed to the operation of the two units, Vicky was concerned that Hospice of the Piedmont might be in danger of moving away from its traditional focus of enabling patients to remain in the setting they consider home — whether it be the family residence, a nursing home or retirement facility.

As 1996 was winding down, a significant decrease in operating revenues was noted, much of it coming from the decrease in number of patients being cared for at home and the increase in late referrals. It was also noted that the budget and staff numbers had been predicated on a patient census of 160, while the census had been wavering for over a year at 130–135. Numerous meetings were held with field staff regarding the need to bring staffing to a more appropriate level; the board named Dick Dershimer to head up a task force on staffing reorganization.

The task force recommendations were announced to an anxious staff in early November. With two previously announced resignations in nursing for unrelated family reasons and five nurses choosing to cut back to four-day weeks, no one in nursing would be laid off; the four patient care teams would be reduced to three; team leader Jean Bradley, RN, would assume the newly created position of assistant director of nursing, absorbing the duties of an eliminated part-time quality assurance nurse and many of the administrative duties previously borne by team leaders; and one social work position and one volunteer coordinator position would be eliminated.

Vicky Todd acknowledged that the staff was not pleased with the proposed plan, but that it was necessary for the Hospice's future. Board members indicated that they, too, had agonized over the situation, but that they realized a plan needed to be implemented by January 1, 1997. In order to clarify the staffing policy going forward, Dick Dershimer presented the following resolution, which was unanimously adopted by the board:

"It is the policy of Hospice of the Piedmont that patient care staffing patterns will be consistent with norms for hospices across the country. Hospice of the Piedmont will strive to maintain case loads that are, on average, at the midpoint of established ranges. It is recognized that acuity and travel time will cause variations in the size of caseloads within Hospice of the Piedmont, and that temporary imbalances may exist due to fluctuations in the average daily census and geographical considerations. Census data and case loads will be evaluated on a quarterly basis to see that appropriate staffing levels are maintained."

While dealing with this staffing issue, Vicky and the board were concerned that the staff's commitment to superior care for patients and their families not be diminished. Happily, the year-end report of the Quality Assurance Committee provided a much-needed affirmation of the staff's ongoing commitment — the patient family surveys continued to be overwhelmingly positive.

Following an early December reception at Church of the Incarnation, planned by hospice volunteers, the fifth Hospice Tree ceremony was held at nearby Fashion Square Mall. Led by chaplains Marvin Barbre and Karl Netting, the ceremony was unusually well attended. The huge tree, erected earlier with the help of hospice volunteers, was filled with lights placed by over 700 persons in memory or in honor of loved ones. In the process, they had contributed a total of $25,000 to the work of Hospice of the Piedmont.

In March 1997, the Inspector General's Office (OIG) of the Department of Health and Human Services announced the extension of Operation Restore Trust (ORT) to include all 50 states. The announcement created considerable concern within the nation's hospices. From a growing number of stories appearing in the national press, it had become obvious that federal auditors were focused on challenging the terminal diagnoses of hospice patients living more than 210 days; and they were recommending that insurance companies handling Medicare claims move to collect reimbursement for challenged claims paid to hospices.

The Hospice of the Florida Suncoast, which was caring for more than 3,000 patients each year, was highlighted in a number of news stories during this time. After scrutinizing a random sample of its patients who had lived more than 210 days, federal auditors said that many of them should never have been admitted to hospice care because a terminal diagnosis was uncertain. About half of these were cancer patients; a smaller number had AIDS. Mary J. Labyak, executive director of the

Hospice of the Florida Suncoast, expressed grave concern over these rulings. "What do you do when people live too long?" she asked. Pointing out that physicians and their dying patients could become hesitant to use hospice services, Labyak related that one of her long-lived patients had told her staff: "I just feel terrible because I am one of those people who cause hospice trouble. I would die if I could but God just won't take me."

Although predicting when someone is going to die is hardly an exact science, it is estimated that at least 85 percent of hospice patients do die within six months, with a small number living beyond 210 days. Terminally ill hospice patients often live longer than expected because of the quality of care they receive. To complicate predicting how long a patient will live, when Medicare regulations for hospice care were first drawn up, nearly all hospice patients had a terminal cancer diagnosis. Today, many other terminal conditions are cared for — including lung and heart disease, AIDS, and Alzheimer's, for which death is more difficult to predict.

Vicky Todd noted in her March 1997 report to the board that future Medicare billing would be based on the patient's zip code, rather than the address of the hospice office. For Hospice of the Piedmont, this would translate into a lower rate of reimbursement for patients living in the more rural parts of its large service area. In discussing the spread of the OIG investigations into all states, Vicky said she would not be surprised to see Hospice of the Piedmont investigated, if for no other reason than its size. Out of a current census of 140, 35 patients had been receiving hospice care for more than 210 days.

At the May 28, 1997, board meeting, Vicky reported that the "length of stay" investigations of the OIG were having a chilling effect on hospice referrals, exacerbated by a new ruling that there would be a financial penalty for physicians who referred "ineligible patients" to hospice programs.

After three very eventful years as president of the board, John F. Harlan completed his term of office in June 1997. John was honored at the July board meeting, not only for his years as president, but for completing his second three-year term as a board member and for the new level of connectedness his experience with the community and the health field had brought to Hospice of the Piedmont. Bruce B. Galloway was elected to succeed John as board president, with Jerry Bailey serving as vice president.

The Balanced Budget Act of 1997 contained a significant restructuring of the Hospice Medicare Benefit periods, allowing for two ninety-day benefit periods, and an unlimited number of sixty-day benefit periods — a change that would benefit some longer-term patients. The change required physician recertification every sixty days but, since patients could be readmitted to hospice in a new sixty-day period at any point, it eliminated the "all or nothing" system hospices had been working under, whereby a patient discharged during the open-ended benefit period could never again be admitted to the Hospice Medicare Benefit.

During the late fall of 1997, Hospice of the Piedmont experienced a serious dip in the patient census — most of it in the number of patients being cared for at home. From a fairly stable census of 135 in November 1996, the number of patients being cared for in November 1997 had declined to 99. In her report to the board, Vicky attributed part of the decline to the establishment of a certified hospice at Augusta Medical Center; for the rest, there was no apparent reason. She also apprised the board that staff members were meeting with a consultant to explore ways of improving communication and support in the hospice working environment.

Vicky concluded her year-end report with the emotional story of one of the staff nurses who had been diagnosed with metastatic cancer. The terminal disease was so advanced that she would not be able to return to work. With her family dependent on her income, she didn't know where to turn. In addition to losing her income, the loss of her health insurance at this point would be a total disaster. Unfortunately, Vicky explained, she had been working only 24 hours a week, making her ineligible for Hospice of the Piedmont's disability insurance, which required a weekly minimum of 30 hours. "Telling her this was one of the hardest things I've ever had to do." As members of the staff learned of the situation and searched for ways they could help, it was suggested that they consider donating up to three days each of their own sick leave. The response was so great that her eligibility for health insurance and payment of her part-time salary could continue for a full year.

The sixth annual Hospice Tree lighting took place on December 2, 1997, with a late afternoon reception at Church of the Incarnation and the lighting ceremony in front of the

Hospice offices on the corner of 29 North and Westfield Road. Robert Van Winkle, a popular local television personality, conducted an on-site interview as the staff and friends of hospice gathered for the impressive ceremony in memory and in honor of loved ones. The 25-foot tree was donated by staff member Patti Gardener Jackson in memory of her mother, Martha Gardner, who had been a Hospice of the Piedmont patient.

In a newsletter article, Vicky characterized 1997 as "tumultuous" — pointing to the tightening of Medicare regulations and significant changes in Medicare reimbursement for hospice care contained in the Budget Reconciliation Bill. "As a result of these and other factors," she said, "we enter 1998 facing the reality of diminished financial resources and the challenge of learning to do more with less. In spite of these challenges, I truly feel optimistic about the future of Hospice of the Piedmont. . . . as we strive to make the essence of hospice care available to all who need and want our care."

As 1998 opened, the patient census remained in the 90's — the lowest level seen in some years. As a result, the operating deficit was growing rapidly and another reorganization became imperative. At the January meeting of the board, the personnel committee recommended the elimination of six to eight positions. At that same meeting, the board learned that Martha Jefferson Hospital was building a primary care office on Route 250 East, at the entrance to Westminster Canterbury of the Blue Ridge, and was offering Hospice of the Piedmont the opportunity of leasing the upper floor of the building, an arrangement that would save approximately $30,000 per year in rent.

A highlight of the spring was the annual conference of the statewide Virginia Association for Hospices held in Charlottesville. After a full year of planning, Hospice of the Piedmont hosted the event at the Omni Charlottesville Hotel. Attracting a record attendance, the conference was acclaimed the most successful in memory, with many kudos given for its organization, the quality of the speakers, and the exceptional hospitality provided by the hospice staff and volunteers.

At the May meeting of the board, Vicky Todd reported that, while the downsizing needed to bring staffing in line with patient census had been very difficult for all, she was confident that the staff was committed to move along in a positive fashion to continue providing superior end-of-life care. Vicky also reported the troubling news that the Medicare intermediary had placed Hospice of the Piedmont on focused medical review. This had resulted from some of the recently submitted patient records being declared ineligible for payment because they did not qualify for the Medicare hospice benefit. She explained that, for the next quarter, it would be necessary to submit some charts of current patients at the intermediary's request, with payment postponed until they had been reviewed. Vicky acknowledged that this had been an extremely trying period for everyone associated with Hospice of the Piedmont.

A few weeks later, the staff was surprised to learn of Vicky Todd's decision to step down as executive director, as of July 2, 1998, and embark on a new path. After twenty years of work in human services, she had decided to act on her increasingly serious interest in horticulture and enroll in a graduate program leading to a Ph.D in that field, with an eventual goal of teaching at the college level.

Citing her strong commitment to education, her grappling with significant changes in the health care system, and her building of bridges to the AIDS community, board president Bruce Galloway wrote: "We salute Vicky for her effective and innovative leadership over the past five years, and wish her all good things as she embarks on this new venture."

❧ *Chapter 9*

LIVING IN THE MIDST OF CHANGE

Following Vicky Todd's resignation, the Board of Directors named longtime board member Jerry Bailey to the position of interim executive director. In order to accept the position, Jerry resigned his membership on the board. Board president Bruce Galloway voiced his appreciation for Jerry's ten years of faithful service and his confidence in Jerry's ability to lead the agency while a new executive director was sought.

In early August 1998, a surveyor from the state made an unannounced visit to perform the annual license renewal audit. Jean Bradley, who had become director of nurses upon Jane Griffith's recent departure, was given high marks for doing an outstanding job in accommodating the surveyor during the lengthy process and keeping disruptions to the rest of the staff at a minimum.

At the very busy August meeting of the board, Frances S. Bonardi, RN, was welcomed to board membership. A longtime friend of hospice, Fran was vice president for operations at Martha Jefferson Hospital, a post she had held since 1986. She was destined to be elected president of Hospice of the Piedmont's board at the completion of Bruce Galloway's term in 1999.

As a beginning point for establishing a search committee for a new executive director, Bruce suggested that board members be appointed first so that interacting with staff could begin as soon as possible. Brooks Marshall, Dick Dershimer, Fran Bonardi, and Bruce Galloway all agreed to serve on the committee, with Dick Dershimer designated as chairman. Decisions on staff representation were postponed for the time being.

Construction of Martha Jefferson Hospital's new office building on Route 250 East got underway during the late summer of 1998. Susan Rives of the board, with major input from senior administrative and clinical staff of hospice, had worked tirelessly with MJH personnel in finalizing the floor plan and all the physical construction and interior details for the upper level to be leased by Hospice of the Piedmont. The new building was expected to be completed in early spring, with an estimated move-in date of March 1, 1999.

In late September 1998, the board received the welcome news that Wellmark, the Medicare intermediary, after reviewing the records of 54 recent patients of Hospice of the Piedmont, was lifting the focused Medicare review, effective October 9, 1998. In addition to affirming better documentation of eligibility for the Hospice Medicare Benefit in these recent patient records, the lifting of the focused review had the practical effect of freeing up payment of a substantial number of Medicare claims that had been held up for months by the review process.

At its October meeting, the board learned that the green light had finally been given for providing a "bridge program" to address the needs of patients who faced limited life expectancy but did not qualify for, or need, the comprehensive services of a Medicare-certified hospice program. After making tentative plans to develop such a support program in late 1997, Hospice of the Piedmont had wisely joined other hospices in seeking legal counsel for officially providing the program and, finally, this answer: Yes, you may offer such a program, provided it is maintained with meticulous recordkeeping as a separate cost center and is funded by community support, with some of Hospice of the Piedmont's fundraising efforts dedicated specifically for the program. The service would use the same volunteer pool as Hospice of the Piedmont; it would coordinate with the attending physician in assessing the emotional, spiritual and practical needs of the patient/family and in determining how the program could help meet those needs. There would be no fee for these services, nor would they replace any fee-based services offered by other agencies. The lawyers involved in providing this counsel also assisted in structuring a separate admissions packet for the program. After careful discussion, the board enthusiastically committed itself to this new initiative for a period of three years and voted to create an advisory council to review its viability on a regular basis. Jerry Bailey announced that staff members Karen Boyle,

RN, and Kerri Thompson, MSW, would lead the effort to launch the *Caring Support* program.

Coming on the heels of the tumultuous times just past, this was a bold and significant act — signaling a determination to return to the roots of hospice care, with its promise not to abandon patients with a limited life expectancy, regardless of whether they were continuing to receive aggressive, life-prolonging treatment, had a terminal diagnosis longer than six months, were previously appropriate for hospice services but had stabilized to the extent that the prognosis was no longer less than six months or, while appropriate for hospice, chose not to enroll in hospice.

In the midst of diminished financial resources, the 1998–1999 edition of the *Dining Around The Area* fundraiser provided a bright spot. Begun in 1989, the annual sale of the booklets, containing coupons for free entrées in some of the area's best restaurants, had shown steady growth, with all proceeds benefitting Hospice of the Piedmont. When this 10th anniversary edition went on sale November 1, 1998, it quickly broke all previous records, selling out completely by the end of December, with sales totaling over $105,000. A tremendous debt of gratitude was acknowledged to the generous restaurant owners who, through this program, were continuing to strengthen Hospice of the Piedmont's ability to provide care for all who needed it, regardless of insurance coverage or financial circumstances.

Another bright spot was the 7th annual Hospice Tree celebration of life, held at Church of the Incarnation on the evening of December 1, 1998. Over 200 persons were in attendance — patient families, staff and friends of Hospice of the Piedmont. After the impressive ceremony and the reception that followed, the tree was moved to the front entrance of the hospice offices where it remained lighted until early January.

Meanwhile, the search committee had interviewed four candidates for the executive director position, with staff representatives given the opportunity to meet with each candidate as well. Subsequently, at an executive session of the board on December 16, 1998, the search committee recommended that Jon Derryberry of Cincinnati, Ohio, be chosen as the new executive director. With extensive experience as the administrator of hospices and nursing home agencies in Ohio, Georgia and South Carolina, Jon was unanimously elected to assume the position, effective January 15, 1999.

In assessing the events of 1998, there is ample evidence that patients and their families had continued to receive excellent care. In spite of fiscal concerns, a decline in patient census and the subsequent staff reductions, patient family satisfaction assessments of the quality of care remained very positive. Along with kudos for the competence and compassion of the clinical staff, there were many expressions of gratitude for the friendship and practical help provided by hospice volunteers.

An article in a newsletter from this period provides a window through which we glimpse something of the significant difference volunteers make in hospice care. The article, entitled "While Others Slept," concerns a Hospice of the Piedmont volunteer with a penchant for going beyond expectations in extending himself to patients and their families. The patient to whom he was assigned had died several nights before and Jean Bradley, RN, who was now the patient care coordinator, had been briefed on the details. The article contains excerpts from a letter Jean wrote to the volunteer just before Christmas, 1998. To ensure privacy, the names of the volunteer, the patient and his wife have been changed:

> *Dear Tom:*
> *I was anxious to know how Ricky's death went and how his wife was doing. What I found out touched me so deeply that I felt the need to write you today to say, 'Thank You.' The time commitment you made by staying with Ricky until the middle of the night when he died, was far beyond any expectation. You have given a most precious gift to Ricky, to Donna, to Hospice, and to our community. Thank you for your example and for reminding me of why I joined Hospice of the Piedmont.*

As the year ended, finance director John Lah resigned in order to accept a similar position at the University of Maryland, where he could be nearer his aging parents. The Board presented John with a gift and a framed certificate of appreciation, citing his exemplary service during a crucial period in Hospice of the Piedmont's history.

Shortly before the arrival of the new executive director in early January, Jerry Bailey was subjected to a good-natured "roast" by the hospice staff, during which he received many accolades for his six-month stint as interim executive director. He received many additional expressions of gratitude at the January meeting of the board and, by unanimous vote, was returned to membership on the board.

In early 1999, the United States Postal Service issued its newest commemorative first-class 33¢ stamp — "in recognition of the more than 3,000 hospices, 25,000 professionals and 100,000 volunteers that have increasingly made hospice the end-of-life choice for Americans." The colorful stamp pictured a butterfly over a home, a symbolic expression of the final stage of life's journey. Locally, the new stamp was unveiled on February 9th at a luncheon hosted by Hospice of the Piedmont in the parish hall of Church of Our Saviour on East Rio Road in Charlottesville. Included among the 70 guests at the luncheon were Charlottesville Postmaster Jimmy Morse; Randy Watts, executive director of the Virginia Association for Hospices; and the executive directors of four area hospices: Jon Derryberry of Hospice of the Piedmont; Patsy Tuffy of Hospice of the Rapidan; Judy Matthews of Hospice of the Shenandoah; and Monica Lincoln of Rockingham Memorial Hospice.

Only a few days before this event, the Virginia House of Delegates passed a bill requiring hospice care coverage in all health insurance or HMO plans in Virginia. The bill passed by a 92–5 vote on January 28, 1999, and was later signed into law by Governor Gilmore.

At the February 17th meeting of the board, the new executive director reported on a meeting with Karen Boyle, RN, and Kerri Thompson, MSW, to discuss the *Caring Support* program the board had asked them to launch. Impressed with the potential for serving terminally ill patients who, for a variety of reasons, were not hospice patients, Jon had approved a continued growth of this program from its present census of 29 to a capacity of 50. Utilizing trained volunteers, social workers and chaplains, the program was structured to furnish practical, emotional and spiritual assistance to these patients and their families and, as previously outlined, would be funded by community support.

The move into the new medical office building on 250 East took place on April 17, 1999. Just off the entrance road to Westminster Canterbury of the Blue Ridge, the lower level of the building was designated for medical offices, with Hospice of the Piedmont leasing the upper level. A well-attended open house, jointly sponsored by Martha Jefferson Hospital and Hospice of the Piedmont, was held at the new office building on the afternoon of June 6th.

At the May 19, 1999 meeting of the board, Jon Derryberry proposed a long-term care (LTC) initiative. Holding that the LTC community was not being given the proper attention and was being severely underserved, he said he had never seen such a potential for growth. He recommended that a consultant be brought on board to develop the LTC plan over the next 90 days. At the end of that period, if the consultant and hospice were in agreement, the position would become full-time. This individual would become the point person for promoting timely referrals of terminally ill patients residing in LTC facilities. Jon reported that he had someone in mind for the position — someone on the staff of a hospice in Georgia with extensive experience in developing LTC relations. With Board approval, Jon invited Sharon Britt, LPN, of Savannah, to assume the position of LTC consultant. Accepting the invitation, Sharon arrived in Charlottesville on June 10, 1999, beginning what was to be an extremely fruitful long-term commitment to Hospice of the Piedmont. Over the coming months, she would be busily engaged in establishing personal relationships with members of the medical community and officials of area LTC facilities — relationships that would increase understanding of the full range of services available through Hospice of the Piedmont and the support it could provide for terminally ill patients in LTC facilities.

On the national scene, some observers were becoming convinced that "Operation Restore Trust," the government's antifraud campaign, was doing more harm than good. With the growing reluctance of physicians to refer, more aggressive treatments, and Medicare's complex rules, referrals to hospice were coming later and later, resulting in a shorter median length of stay for hospice patients. One was left to wonder if the terminally ill were receiving the services intended by Congress when the Hospice Benefit was included in Medicare or if, instead of meeting the needs of dying patients, late referrals were creating more stress in these patients, their caregivers and their physicians. Meanwhile, the average daily census of Hospice of the Piedmont was holding at 65.

In mid-August 1999, after a brief tenure as executive director, Jon Derryberry left Hospice of the Piedmont, moving to the west coast to work as a hospice consultant. The board named Jean Bradley, RN, to serve as interim director until a new executive director was in place and elected Fran Bonardi to succeed Bruce Galloway, whose three-year term as president of the board was expiring. As Jean and Fran were assured of the wholehearted support of the Board, Bruce received many expressions of gratitude for the extraordinary leadership he had provided during a very challenging time in Hospice of the Piedmont's history.

The board and staff were saddened to learn of the death of Dr. George Cooper, III, on November 6, 1999, at the age of 91. The distinguished radiologist had been a guiding light in the founding of Hospice of the Piedmont in 1980. As the first president of the board, he had worked closely with Adge Coburn in the formative stages of the organization and remained vitally interested in its progress through the years. He was fond of referring to Adge as "the engine and instigator" of Hospice of the Piedmont but, as Adge was always quick to respond, Dr. Cooper's contribution to the successful establishment of Hospice of the Piedmont was enormous.

During this time, marked by so many changes, Karen Boyle, RN, a longtime staff member who had served as field nurse and liaison nurse for the inpatient unit at UVa, and was instrumental in launching the new *Caring Support* program for non-hospice patients, became the liaison nurse for the expanding palliative care program at UVa, and Helen Destrempes, BSW, who had served both as volunteer coordinator and field social worker, retired after nine years on staff. There were new additions as well, including Senior Accountant Randy Rudolph and Accounts Assistant Joyce Baldwin, both of whom became very popular and respected members of the staff.

Looking back on this period of its history, one is struck once more by Hospice of the Piedmont's unwavering commitment to provide superior care for its patients and families, and its ability to survive and cope with the many changes that came its way — including the inevitable departures of some very valued staff members.

The fall newsletter in 1999 featured a timely article by Interim Director Jean Bradley entitled, "Living in the Midst of Change." Bidding a fond farewell to some extremely dedicated staff members, including those listed above, and welcoming the new members to staff, she wrote: "Change is at the heart of what we do at Hospice of the Piedmont — both in the lists of patients and families we serve and in the dedicated staff members who deliver that service. It is inevitable and, although we never grow completely used to it, we learn to cope with it. In recent months, some extremely dedicated staff members have left us — all for good reason, but their departure leaves an empty place in our hearts, and we will miss them profoundly. . . . As we bid them adieu, we welcome new staff members who have chosen to commit themselves to this work. . . . Welcome, friends — you have big shoes to fill!"

And, somehow, fill them, they did!

The 8th Hospice Tree celebration of life was held on December 7, 1999, at Church of Our Saviour, its sanctuary overflowing with Hospice staff, volunteers, patient families and community friends of Hospice. Following a meditation by Chaplain Karl Netting and a moving candlelighting ceremony led by Bereavement Counselor Beth Smith, the tree was lighted — each of its clear bulbs placed there in memory of a loved one, or in honor of a special person still living. After a reception hosted by Hospice volunteers, the tree was taken to the new Hospice offices, where it remained lighted until early January 2000 and the beginning of a new era in the history of Hospice of the Piedmont.

Chapter 10

BACK TO THE FUTURE

A s the search for a new executive director got underway
during the late summer of 1999, the board was determined
to find an experienced hospice administrator who could meet
several key criteria. The ideal person would have a solid grasp
of the history and philosophy of hospice care, a passionate
commitment to deliver that care to the terminally ill, and the
management skills to lead Hospice of the Piedmont into a
growing future. Confident that it had found such a person, the
search committee recommended Roberta M. White, MSW,
as the new executive director. After hearing the details of her
experience, the board enthusiastically concurred, electing her
by unanimous vote. Roberta assumed her new position on
February 14, 2000.

An experienced and distinguished hospice administrator,
Roberta came to Hospice of the Piedmont from Paramus,
New Jersey, where she had been director of hospice for Valley
Home Care, Inc., since 1995. Prior to that time, she was a
hospice and home care social worker in a community hospice
in Westwood, New Jersey, and manager of social services for
Valley Home Care in Paramus. The creator of the Valley Home

Care Ethics Advisory Committee, Roberta was recognized nationally as an expert in establishing hospice and home care ethics committees. Her professional affiliations included the Board of Directors of the Hospice Network of New Jersey, the Hospice Association of America, for which she was regional faculty presenter on ethics, and the New Jersey Hospice and Palliative Care Organization, which she had chaired in 1999.

At a staff meeting prior to Roberta's arrival, Jean Bradley was honored for her leadership as interim executive director during the previous six months. In a surprise tribute, the staff presented her with a number of gifts and unveiled a huge greeting card, inscribed with personal messages of gratitude for her exceptional service. A valued member of staff since 1992, Jean had served with distinction in the area of quality assurance and, more recently, as a patient care coordinator. One of Roberta's first acts as executive director was to elevate her to the position of director of nursing. With Jean's promotion and the retirement of her colleague Mary Miller, both patient care coordinator positions became vacant, opening the way for outstanding field nurses Theresa O'Brien and Jenny Tompkins to assume those roles.

As we shall see in the following chapters, three major initiatives were mounted during the opening years of Roberta's tenure, focused on meeting unique needs — *Transitions*, a free service for pre-hospice patients; the opening of *Hospice House* for those unable to remain at home during the final stages of their illness; and *Journeys*, an art therapy and seasonal camp program to support children and young people in dealing with the loss of a loved one. Each of these initiatives was destined to thrive and become integral parts of Hospice of the Piedmont's end-of-life care in central Virginia.

During most of 2000, the average daily patient census remained in the mid 80's, with a disturbing number of patients being referred too late to receive the full benefits of hospice care. Roberta's early reports to the board addressed this concern, and the obvious need for increased efforts to both educate and encourage physicians to refer sooner and to help patients and their families make the choice for hospice. As a beginning, she authorized the purchase of extensive marketing and public relations material for use in addressing these needs — educational brochures, print ads, and radio and TV spots, all emphasizing the real issues people face when nearing the end of life, and Hospice of the Piedmont's ability to make a profound difference by sharing the journey with them and their families.

The record of Roberta's first year as executive director is filled with a dizzying number of actions she initiated to ensure a staff committed to the highest level of patient care, and programs that, more often than not, exceeded the requirements of the Hospice Medicare Benefit. In many ways, it was a time of return and recommitment to the roots of hospice care. Looking back on that first year, Roberta acknowledged that the management staff "must have felt like they lived a lifetime in one year as we redesigned services and programs to meet our patient's and family's needs and dedicated ourselves to having exceptional staff at the bedside."

If the staff anticipated a slowing down of the search for more effective ways of educating the public on hospice care and for more innovative ways of meeting the changing needs of patients and their loved ones, they were mistaken — the passionate search would continue unabated.

In April 2000, the Office of the Inspector General (OIG) issued an advisory opinion dealing with the provision of certain types of free care to patients who did not meet the criteria for admission to hospice services. In the advisory opinion, OIG expressed several concerns, including its determination that the benefits of such a program " . . . are provided at least in part to induce patients to obtain hospice care from the Hospice at the appropriate time." Additionally, the advisory raised concerns about these free services being provided in nursing homes, although the services did not duplicate any nursing home services. These and other OIG concerns had implications for *Caring Support*, a pre-hospice program sponsored by Hospice of the Piedmont. As a consequence, the program was discontinued in the nursing homes, the practice of using the salaried chaplains was suspended, and a call went out for volunteer chaplains to complement the other volunteers in the program.

Meanwhile, *Transitions*, a volunteer-based pre-hospice program that retained many of the best features of the *Caring Support* program, had received tacit approval in an OIG advisory opinion. The decision was made to sponsor the *Transitions* program and transfer the remaining *Caring Support* clients into it. The impetus for sponsoring *Transitions* grew out of the awareness of that significant number of persons with a terminal diagnosis who, for a variety of reasons, may not be eligible for hospice care or ready to choose hospice care and find themselves without any meaningful support. Designed by veteran hospice professional Peter Briguglio, MA, *Transitions* would be offered without charge and provide case management for clients with a life-limiting illness and a prognosis of about one year. Eligibility for the program would not be contingent on whether or not the client was receiving curative treatment. Clients would be supported by caring, trained and experienced volunteers providing everything from companionship, to rides to medical appointments, to linking to community services, to respite for family members and caregivers, to help with advanced directives to spell out to the medical community what interventions were wanted or not wanted. Peter Briguglio agreed to spend December 10 and 11 at Hospice of the Piedmont to personally provide intensive training for implementing this new program. It was agreed that the program would be phased in gradually as volunteers were trained and the community became more aware of this new resource in end-of-life care.

Perhaps the most unexpected event of the opening months of Roberta's tenure was the closing of the hospice inpatient unit at UVa in the early summer of 2000. With the 1995 contract between Hospice and UVa for the Center for Hospice and Palliative Care up for renegotiation, Roberta and the board felt constrained to close the unit. The difficult decision took a number of factors into account — the unit's high operating cost, the difficulty of finding and retaining adequate staffing, the lack of interdisciplinary care so vital to hospice care, and a drifting away from the basic hospice model of enabling patients to remain at home, or wherever they call home, with support, not in an institutional setting.

With the closing of the dedicated hospice unit at UVa, it was agreed that the Palliative Care Unit would be designated as the place of choice for incoming hospice patients and, if there were no available beds, the patients would be placed on medical surgical floors while being followed by the hospice team. The hospice volunteers would continue working in the Palliative Care Unit.

The recent "focused medical review" for overutilization of inpatient care for hospice patients had taken its toll on the financial reserves of the agency. In addition to her ongoing commitment to excellence in caring for patients and their family members, Roberta focused on strategies to strengthen the fiscal health of Hospice of the Piedmont. Billing specialist Debbie Johnson, who had worked effectively with accountant Randy Rudolph in compiling the detailed financial data needed for the 1999–2000 accounting audit, was promoted to manager of billing and information services in recognition of her demonstrated ability to organize and plan for both of these needs within the agency. She was cited for being "single minded in her pursuit of accurate and timely billing while struggling with the problems Medicare poses every day." In early September 2000, Sam Morgan, CPA, was hired as chief financial officer, bringing a strong background in healthcare finance. Unaware that he had just received the Muncie Award from the Health Finance Management Association, he was completely surprised when Debbie Johnson presented the award to him on his first day with hospice. Other staff additions during this period included Rose Thomas to support Debbie in the complex, time-consuming clinical documentation needed for Medicare billing.

On Our Own Terms, a series on dying produced by Bill Moyers, was televised on PBS on four successive evenings in September 2000. Containing the stories of dying persons, their families and caregivers, the six-hour production centered on the growing struggle in the care of terminally ill patients to balance medical intervention with comfort and humanity. Although hospice professionals had a mixed reaction to the way hospice was portrayed, the series generated a great deal of thought and conversation about how we care for the dying in America.

Explaining that he tackled the experience of death because of the relevance of the issue for the aging baby boomers, Moyers acknowledged that his work on this series had changed him as a human being. He found himself astonished by how much people were willing to share concerning the "supremely intimate" experience of death and found that he was helped in caring for his own mother by those he interviewed for the series. His personal connection deepened significantly when, on the day filming began, his mother died.

In the fall of 2000, the development subcommittee of the board, chaired by Pat Coffey, began its work of establishing a plan for a residential hospice house. With the promise of support for such a facility by an anonymous donor, discussions centered on the need for a feasibility study to determine the degree of community support for a sizeable capital campaign.

Meanwhile, the need for a comprehensive strategic plan for the agency had become crucial and proposals for leading a strategic planning process were sought from a number of experienced hospice consultants. In the end, the proposal of John Sheetz was accepted, with plans to begin the process in the first quarter of 2001.

Some valued staff members left Hospice of the Piedmont during this time — most of them moving to other locations in Virginia and beyond: Pam Kimmel, who through the years had served in various administrative roles, including office manager and HR manager; chaplain Karl Netting who, after six years of commuting from Richmond, accepted a like position with a Richmond hospice; Beth Smith, a bereavement coordinator, who moved with her minister husband to his new pastorate in Richmond; and Kate Fraleigh, RN, who moved to San Francisco, where she hoped to continue her work in hospice care. New additions to staff during this period included Katie Heidingsfelger, LCSW, Donna Moyer, RN, and Sara Kassel, LCSW, who accepted the position of director of counseling and social work.

One morning in late October, shortly after the mail was delivered, an unusually loud and joyful sound emanated from Roberta's office. She held in her hands the just-opened letter from a local law firm, conveying the deep appreciation of their client for the compassionate care the clinical staff and volunteers of Hospice of the Piedmont had provided during the final months of her life. Enclosed was a check for a very substantial bequest from her estate, with the stipulation that it be added to the endowment fund to ensure such care for future patients. Roberta and her staff were overwhelmed by this dear lady's affirmation of the compassionate care she had received, and her generous bequest to provide it for others. Coming when it did, after the relative turbulence and uncertainty of the recent past, the serendipitous event was a humbling reminder of both the privilege and the importance of "sharing the journey" with the terminally ill and their loved ones.

A busy December included the ninth annual Hospice Tree celebration at Church of the Incarnation and Peter Briguglio's two-day visit to provide on-site training for *Transitions*. Trish Gomez, an experienced LCSW with a strong clinical background and a long involvement in hospice, was designated as the case manager for the new program, which would become a major source of support for pre-hospice clients and their families throughout the area.

The journey back to the future had begun.

Chapter 11
WHEN THE WORLD CHANGED

The terrorist attack of 2001 left a gnawing sense of insecurity in the national psyche and ultimately triggered two wars. Attacks of Afghan targets by U.S. air and naval forces with British support began on October 7, 2001, with U.S. B-52 bombing attacks in Afghanistan commencing on November 1. Some 16 months later, on March 18, 2003, acting on a belief in some circles that terrorism and its sponsors could not be eradicated as long as Saddam Hussein was in power, American and British troops invaded Iraq, intent on removing him. The invasion was only the beginning of a protracted struggle that would, along with the continuing conflict in Afghanistan, exact a terrible toll in human lives.

Yet, as the early months of 2001 unfolded, there was little reason to expect such dire events. As far as Hospice of the Piedmont was concerned, there was strong evidence that the agency was entering a period of stability. Under Roberta White's leadership, there was renewed commitment to the historic roots of hospice care, with its attention to innovative pain/symptom control and support of the social, emotional and spiritual needs of patients and their families. Plans were underway for individualized orientation of new staff, a preceptor program, and the provision of ongoing education and training opportunities. The appointment of directors for nursing, social work, counseling, and quality assurance was providing strong guidance for the staff and setting high standards for patient care and family support. In addition, there was a growing utilization of volunteers in a number of areas, including *Transitions*, *Journeys*, clerical support, community outreach and education — a daily reminder that volunteers continued to be "the heart of hospice."

Soon after her arrival in late 2000, Sara Kassel, the new director of counseling and social work, with extensive experience in bereavement services for children, began working with art therapist Stephanie Wilson in designing the fledgling *Journeys* bereavement program and accepting its early referrals. The decision to offer the innovative program as a public service had grown out of the recognition that children and adolescents are often the forgotten grievers.

Utilizing individual counsel and age-appropriate support groups, the program was designed to provide children and teens with a safe place to express the grief, anger, and fear related to loss — thereby enhancing the development of important coping skills. Through supportive activities, they would learn that they were not alone and that their feelings were normal. Registered art therapists and trained volunteers would use art and other creative means to help them express their inner feelings, while parents and guardians would meet with bereavement counselors for support in living with their own loss and for guidance in supporting their grieving children.

Along the way, the provision of seasonal bereavement camps would become a popular feature of the *Journeys* program — both day and overnight experiences. Typical camp activities would include art/expressive activity, sharing time, creating memories, recreational activities suited to the season, and a closing ceremony. Parents would be encouraged to participate in a support group and in the memorial ceremony at each seasonal camp.

As part of Hospice of the Piedmont's commitment to the community, *Journeys* services would be made available to schools, community groups and the general public, including grief support groups facilitated by bereavement counselors and/or registered art therapists for agencies or groups working with children and teens.

Stephanie Wilson's availability for work in the program was somewhat limited because of family commitments and, as the program began to grow, a search began for an additional board certified art therapist. The search led to the hiring of Kacie Woodard Karafa in June 2001.

Early referrals to the Journeys bereavement program came from the two local hospitals, a home care agency and a Head Start program that referred a family of three children who had lost their mother a year before and were living with their grandmother, who had been diagnosed as terminally ill with about a year to live. Hospice of the Piedmont was able

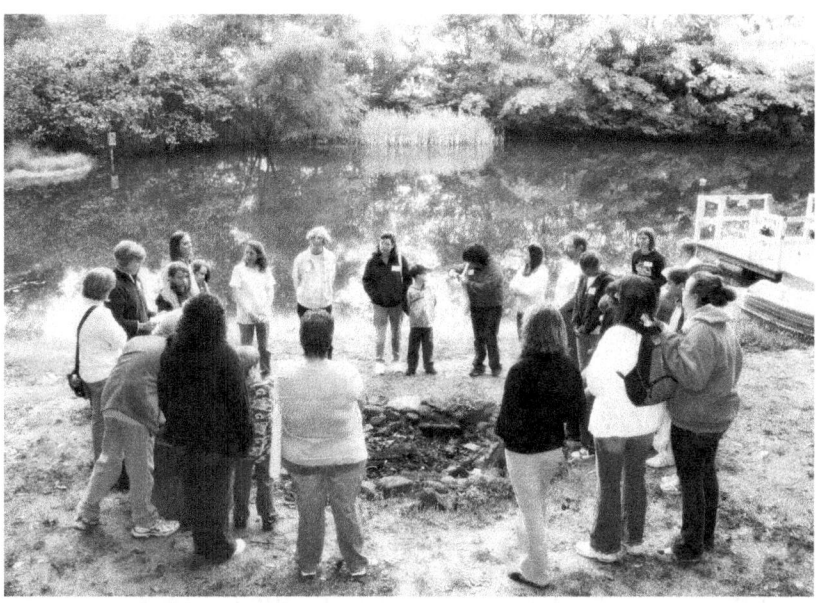

Closing ceremony at a Journeys bereavement camp.

to provide *Transitions* for the grandmother and *Journeys* to support the children.

By early summer, the strategic planning process was well underway with consultant John Sheetz, who was leading a series of meetings with a committee comprising board members and senior management staff. Under John's guidance, tentative statements of mission, vision, values and goals were drafted for board consideration.

During this same period, Charlie Witzleben of Chapel Hill, North Carolina, was employed to conduct a feasibility study for a capital campaign to fund the establishment of a hospice house and provide sufficient endowment to ensure its long-term viability. Mr. Witzleben had an impressive track record as a development consultant for a variety of clients throughout the country and had recently completed the planning and successful execution of a sizeable capital campaign for a hospice in Savannah, Georgia. In early April, Roberta and the directors of finance and development met with Charlie to begin work on the feasibility study. In the weeks following, the group developed a case statement and a list of potential donors, with whom Charlie would meet during June and July.

Staff changes during this period included the promotion of Barbara Moorhead to the position of volunteer manager, with primary responsibility for the *Transitions* program. Faith Burch, BSW, joined the staff as the new coordinator for *Transitions*.

On July 16, 2001, the hospice inpatient unit at Martha Jefferson Hospital was closed. Roberta explained that this was a difficult but unavoidable decision based on the inability to hire and retain nurses for the unit, combined with the increasing cost to hospice as improved control of pain and symptoms resulted in fewer admissions to the unit. It was agreed that Brenda Welch, RN, and Diane Kudrow, RN, would continue to act as nurse liaisons between the hospital and hospice. The same contractual arrangement that had been made with UVa over a year before would apply at Martha Jefferson Hospital, with patients being followed by the hospice team and hospice volunteers.

Tuesday, September 11, 2001, began routinely enough at the offices of Hospice of the Piedmont — the telephones ringing as usual; two out-of-town auditors at work on the annual financial audit; the clinical staff preparing to get on the road to see patients; eight UVa student nurses and their instructor getting directions to the room reserved for their use, and some volunteers arriving to prepare a large mailing. "Good morning, how are you? — "Beautiful day" — "Is there some coffee in the kitchen?" — "The copier needs a new ink cartridge." All very routine — but soon you knew it was a day you would remember in detail for the rest of your life . . . much like the day President Kennedy was assassinated in Dallas — this day when a sudden terrorist attack took the lives of some 3,000 persons.

You would remember it – the U. S. commercial airliners used as missiles of destruction: an American Airlines Boeing 767 plowing into the North Tower of New York's World Trade Center at 8:46 a.m.; a second American Airlines Boeing 767 hitting the South Tower at 9:03; an American Airlines Boeing 757 crashing into the Pentagon at 9:37; and a United Airlines Boeing 757, thought to be headed for the White House or Capitol, crashing in a field in Pennsylvania, at 10:03, after a group of passengers had overcome the hijackers.

You would remember what you were doing when you heard the first news bulletins on an office radio and how, instinctively, you reached for the telephone to call your spouse. You would remember how quickly the news spread through the building and how those around you reacted. You would remember making your way to the overflowing conference room where someone had tuned in the local network affiliate on the TV normally used for educational videos. You would remember the shock of knowing your country was being attacked and the looks of disbelief on the faces of those around you. You would remember the groans of sorrow as the majestic towers began to crumble, and the quiet tears that could no longer be restrained as the shocking tragedy played out on the conference room television screen and the nation wondered if there was more yet to come. You would remember.

In her board report a week later, Roberta remembered:

"Like the whole world, Hospice was overwhelmed on Tuesday when we heard the news of the terrorist attack. We have staff, patients and families who have family members or friends in New York City and Washington, D.C. . . . The Hospice staff made us proud. Their first concern was for their fellow workers, visitors, students and the patients and families. Our nurses and social workers visited and comforted the patients who had been waiting to hear about loved ones and the Journeys program has been in touch with area schools to offer bereavement support and counseling to the children affected in any way... Sharon Britt was going to the Disney Institute for Health Care Services in Orlando and Dr. John Lanham, our volunteer Medical Director since 1988, was scheduled to attend the Palliative Care Certification training for physicians in San Francisco.

John was understandably uneasy about flying from Dulles the day after the attacks. As it turned out, all domestic flights were cancelled. We are continuing to reach out to our patients and bereaved families in any way possible."

Following the resignation of pharmacist Laura Irwin in October, Bill McCoy was hired. Bill brought many years of clinical pharmacy and compounding experience to the position, as well as a background in pharmacy management. Under his leadership, plans for Hospice of the Piedmont's own pharmacy would go forward, resulting in significant savings in providing patient prescriptions and, through his expertise as a compounding pharmacist, many innovative approaches to symptom control.

At the November board meeting, Charlie Witzleben presented a positive feasibility report based on 36 completed interviews and Roberta reported on the continuing search for land on which to build the proposed Hospice House. The lack of infrastructure and the resulting limitation on the maximum number of occupants allowed was a real problem in Albemarle County, while the cost of suitable acreage in the city of Charlottesville seemed prohibitive.

The year ended with a total of 650 patients having been cared for; some 727 persons also received bereavement support from social workers and from bereavement groups led by chaplains Katha Bollfrasse and Tony Perrino throughout the service area. The average daily patient census had topped

100 and was continuing to rise. Referrals to the pre hospice *Transitions* program were growing and, in addition to three age-appropriate support groups, the *Journeys* program was becoming active in area schools, where services could be provided while a child was still in school.

The Hospice Tree ceremony drew an unusually large attendance, as the community affirmed a special need for this traditional event — remembering both their own loved ones and those unknown to them who had perished on 9/11, the day the world was changed.

Chapter 12

THE JOURNEY TO 501 PARK STREET

It was early afternoon on September 28, 1999, when the middle-aged man pulled off the highway, reached for his car phone and placed a call to Hospice of the Piedmont — something he had been intending to do for some time. With interim director Jean Bradley unavailable at that moment, the receptionist routed the call to me. The caller, a recent transplant from the west coast, had a story to tell and an offer to make.

After the caller introduced himself, the conversation went something like this:

CALLER

"Does your hospice have any plans for a hospice house in the near future?"

HAYNES

"It's certainly a dream of ours — something we intend to pursue as soon as possible. Unfortunately, we don't

have an executive director at the moment and feel we can't move forward in planning for a hospice house until new leadership is in place. It's going to require a sizeable capital campaign."

CALLER
"Well, let me tell you why I asked. My mother was living in Florida several years ago when she was diagnosed with a terminal illness. She spent her final weeks in a wonderful hospice house in Stuart, Florida. The care she received there was unbelievable and I made a promise to myself that, when I was able, I would honor my mother's memory by helping my community have a facility like that."

As our conversation was drawing to a close, he asked if I could arrange for an appropriate group to meet at his home to discuss the matter further. And so it was that, on a morning three days later, four of us gathered at Peter Licata's home outside of Charlottesville — interim executive director Jean Bradley, board vice president Jerry Bailey, chairman of the executive director search committee Dick Dershimer, and I. We spent some time briefing Peter and his wife, Elaine, on our need for a hospice house and the difference it would make to the growing number of terminally ill patients we were seeing who had no caregiver or whose loved ones were unable to provide safe and adequate care during the final stage of their illness. It was noted that the continued influx of retirement-age persons to the area, combined with the aging of the resident Baby Boomer generation, was making the need for a hospice house even more critical. After brainstorming some ideas for finding a suitable location for the new facility, the meeting ended with assurances of substantial support from this new friend of Hospice of the Piedmont.

The Board was informed of this turn of events and, after animated discussion, new board president Fran Bonardi agreed to make personal contact with Peter Licata to convey appreciation for his generous offer and to assure him of our interest in pursuing the dream of a hospice house as soon as possible. The journey to 501 Park Street had begun.

In considering the ideal location for a hospice house, the initial thinking tended to focus on a quiet rural setting away from "the maddening crowd." Indeed, by the time new executive director Roberta White arrived, on February 14, 2000, several areas outside Charlottesville had been pinpointed as possible locations. Roberta and the board found Albemarle County officials most helpful and sympathetic but, as previously noted, the search for such a setting would, in the end, prove fruitless because of the lack of affordable property, zoning restrictions and the absence of sewer and water required for such a facility.

Then, quite unexpectedly, it was learned that Rosewood Manor, an established assisted living facility in Charlottesville, was for sale.

Only blocks away from downtown Charlottesville, Rosewood Manor was the antithesis of a quiet pastoral setting. The large turn-of-the-century house faced historic Park Street, down which hundreds of people drove each day on their way to and from work, business appointments or shopping and entertainment on the Downtown Mall. It hardly seemed the ideal location for a hospice house — at least that was the initial reaction. But, gradually, the realization grew that having this very special facility at the center of the city's life was as it should be. Hospice care was about *living* — about enhancing the quality of *life* — about keeping the promise made early on by Cicely Saunders: "You matter because you are you. You matter to the last moment of your life, and we will do all we can, not only to help you die peacefully, but to live (fully) until you die." The conviction grew that 501 Park Street was, indeed, the right location.

Documents archived at the Albemarle Charlottesville Historical Society trace the long history of the house at 501 Park Street. James E. Irvine purchased the lot on the west side of Park Street from J. D. Watson in 1903 and built "the large Queen Anne House" in 1904. The house is described as "a handsome example of the Victorian Style with Colonial detailing, a frequent combination in pre-World War I Charlottesville." Special mention is made of the "handsome Doric columned Colonial Revival veranda with a rounded corner" gracing the front of the house.

James E. Irvine was born in 1865 in Augusta County. He moved to Charlottesville in 1883 and, after working for some time in clothing businesses, spent over thirty years operating his own clothing establishment on Main Street. In

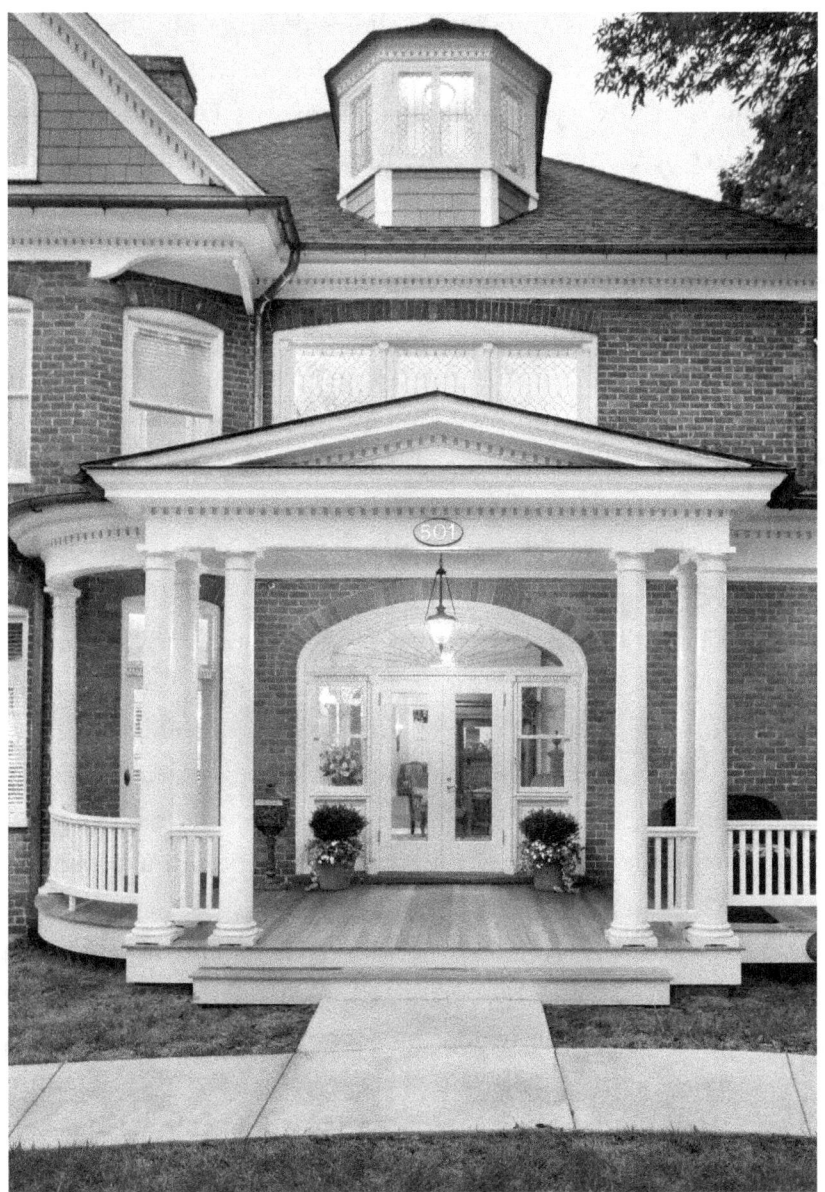

Hospice House — "on sacred ground."

later years, he was engaged in the real estate and insurance business. Mr. Irvine was very active in the community, serving on the City Council, the Board of Directors of the Chamber of Commerce, in the Rotary Club, and as director of the Y.M.C.A. and an elder in the Presbyterian Church. He and his wife, Henrietta Sterrett Irvine, were married in 1892 and had four children — the last one born in June, 1904, the year the house was completed.

The house remained in the Irvine family until 1953, when James Irvine's son John sold the property to G. Morris. His widow, Rachel Morris, used the property as a boarding house for a time before selling it to Michelle Cormier. After continuing to run the boarding house for several years, she conveyed the property to Sameer and Virginia Tahboub in 1982. The following year, after some interior renovation, the Tahboubs opened the house as "a nursing or convalescent home for elderly adults" that, for the next seventeen years, would be known as Rosewood Manor. And now the Tahboubs were building a larger assisted living facility near Charlottesville's Senior Center and the historic house was for sale once more.

Following a ruling by the city that establishment of a hospice house would be permitted at 501 Park Street under the same R-3 zoning and "nursing or convalescent home for elderly adults" designation that had been in effect for Rosewood Manor, the Board of Directors authorized the purchase of the property and, on May 15, 2002, Hospice of the Piedmont became its new owners.

Early on, the Board of Directors approved an ad hoc "Building Task Force Committee" composed of incoming board president Jeanette Lancaster, board member, Peter Licata, board treasurer Rob Freer, board realtor Pat Coffey, executive director Roberta White, and chief financial officer Sam Morgan. Charged with the task of responding to the various issues involved in transforming this historic residence into an exceptional hospice house, the committee undertook the task of finding an outstanding architect to design and produce the schematic plans for the total renovation of the house, and a premier construction firm to review the schematics, develop a line item budget and execute the extensive renovation. After a careful search, the architectural firm of Bruce R. Wardell & Associates and the construction firm of Alexander-Nicholson, Inc. were chosen for this important work. When the line item budget was in hand, the Board of Directors proceeded to approve the launch of a $2,675,000 "Sharing the Journey Campaign" to cover the purchase, expansion and renovation of the home, and provide capital for the new facility's first year of operation. A future $3,000,000 endowment campaign was also projected to ensure the ongoing viability of the hospice house.

The "Sharing the Journey Campaign" faced the formidable challenges of the national sense of insecurity following 9/11, wars in Afghanistan and Iraq and a sharp decline of the stock market that decimated the portfolios of many who would otherwise have been expected to make major gifts. Before approaching foundations, businesses and the general public for support, 100% of the board and staff made commitments to the campaign, pledging an impressive total of $602,861 to be paid over three years.

On May 30, 2002, a proposal was submitted to the Perry Foundation for a challenge grant to be matched during the two-year advance phase of the Sharing the Journey Campaign. Throughout Hospice of the Piedmont's history, this local foundation had provided significant support and, once again, its response was generous. In a letter dated July 17, 2002, Roberta White was informed that the Perry Foundation's Board of Trustees had approved a four-year challenge grant of $200,000 that Hospice of the Piedmont would be required to match by December 1, 2003, through individual and corporate gifts raised after the date of the grant proposal. On December 20, 2002, in a letter to Francis H. Fife, president of the Perry Foundation, Roberta was able to inform the foundation that the matching conditions had been met with additional gifts of $204,000. With the inclusion of the Perry Foundation grant, total commitments to The Sharing the Journey Campaign" had reached a total of $1,140,841. In her letter, Roberta wrote: "We are very grateful to you and the Perry Foundation for your continued support of our work with the terminally ill and their families in this area. During all of our twenty-two year history, the foundation has been there for us and words cannot adequately express our appreciation."

The official launching of the quiet phase of the campaign took place on May 27, 2003, at a tented dinner on the grounds of Peter and Elaine Licata's home. The event was attended by honorary campaign chairperson Sissy Spacek, her husband, Jack Fisk, and 84 guests who were briefed on plans for the future Hospice House and the capital campaign to make it possible. In spite of the faltering economy, it was hoped that significant support would be forthcoming from the carefully chosen guest list — hopes that, with one major exception, were not realized.

One of the highlights of the campaign was the successful effort to secure a sizeable challenge grant from the prestigious Kresge Foundation, headquartered in Troy, Michigan. With the encouragement of development consultant Charles Witzleben, plans were made to go through the demanding grant process required by this foundation. One of the major foundations accepting proposals for "brick and mortar" projects, Kresge grants tended to be completion challenge grants, i.e., grants paid only after the rest of the campaign goal had been successfully attained — a practice that encouraged new donors and expansion of the agency's donor base going forward.

A letter of inquiry to the foundation was followed by a "pre-application visit" to Kresge headquarters on June 25, 2003, by Roberta and board president Jeanette Lancaster, dean of the UVa School of Nursing. With the encouragement of foundation officials, a proposal for a $250,000 completion grant was submitted in mid-July and approved by the Kresge board on December 10, 2003. In order to receive the completion challenge grant, Hospice of the Piedmont was given a deadline of August 31, 2004, to reach a challenge goal of $871,261 — the additional commitments needed to bring the $2,675,000 Sharing the Journey Campaign within $250,000 of successful completion.

Thanks to the generosity of additional area foundations, business organizations and other supporters of hospice care, the challenge goal was met ahead of deadline with the $250,000 completion challenge grant from the Kresge Foundation awarded in early August, 2004. By the end of the successful campaign, a grand total of $2,703,308 in cash and pledges had been received from 27 foundations, 40 business entities, churches and civic clubs, and 657 generous individuals. Honoring requests for anonymity, major donors to the campaign were gratefully acknowledged on an impressive marble plaque at Hospice House.

As the "Sharing the Journey Campaign" was underway, a careful demolition was taking place inside 501 Park Street, in preparation for a creative reworking of its interior spaces for its new role. When the total renovation was complete, the house would include comfortable areas on each floor for visiting families and friends, a kitchen and dining room, and eight private rooms, each with its own bathroom. A commercial elevator would service an admission office on the lower level and the two patient floors above. The top floor, accessed by stairs, would contain a comfortable lounge and a small meditation room for the use of visiting families.

The renovation of the house took place over a full year from November 2003 to November 2004, when the first patients were received. "During that time," Roberta observed, "every person who had a part in bringing the house to life felt they were on 'sacred ground.' We felt at every turn the great respect and pride of our workmen, architects, staff and community in the act of creating a dignified, aesthetically pleasing, and peaceful setting for the dying."

When it was done, the renovated house was beautiful, inside and out. With its brickwork repointed, its wraparound porch rebuilt, its leaded glass and millwork restored and its wood trim freshly painted, it looked absolutely reborn. Walking through the wide entrance door, one encountered the authentic style of a stately 1900 family home, its beautifully appointed parlor to one side, its striking stairway to the other. Among the many accolades received by Hospice of the Piedmont and architects Bruce R. Wardell and Kurt Keesecker was a Preservation Award For Historic Building Rehabilitation from the City of Charlottesville's Board of Architectural Review

While such expressions of approval were gratifying, an important question had yet to be answered: had the dream that motivated the telephone call in 1999 and energized the board, staff and volunteers of Hospice of the Piedmont during this five-year journey to 501 Park Street become a reality? The dream had centered on providing a quiet and peaceful haven for patients unable to remain in their own homes during the final weeks of their lives; a homelike, non-institutional setting where families could deal with end-of-life issues; where family devotion could be affirmed, estrangements overcome, and final goodbyes spoken. Did we get it right?

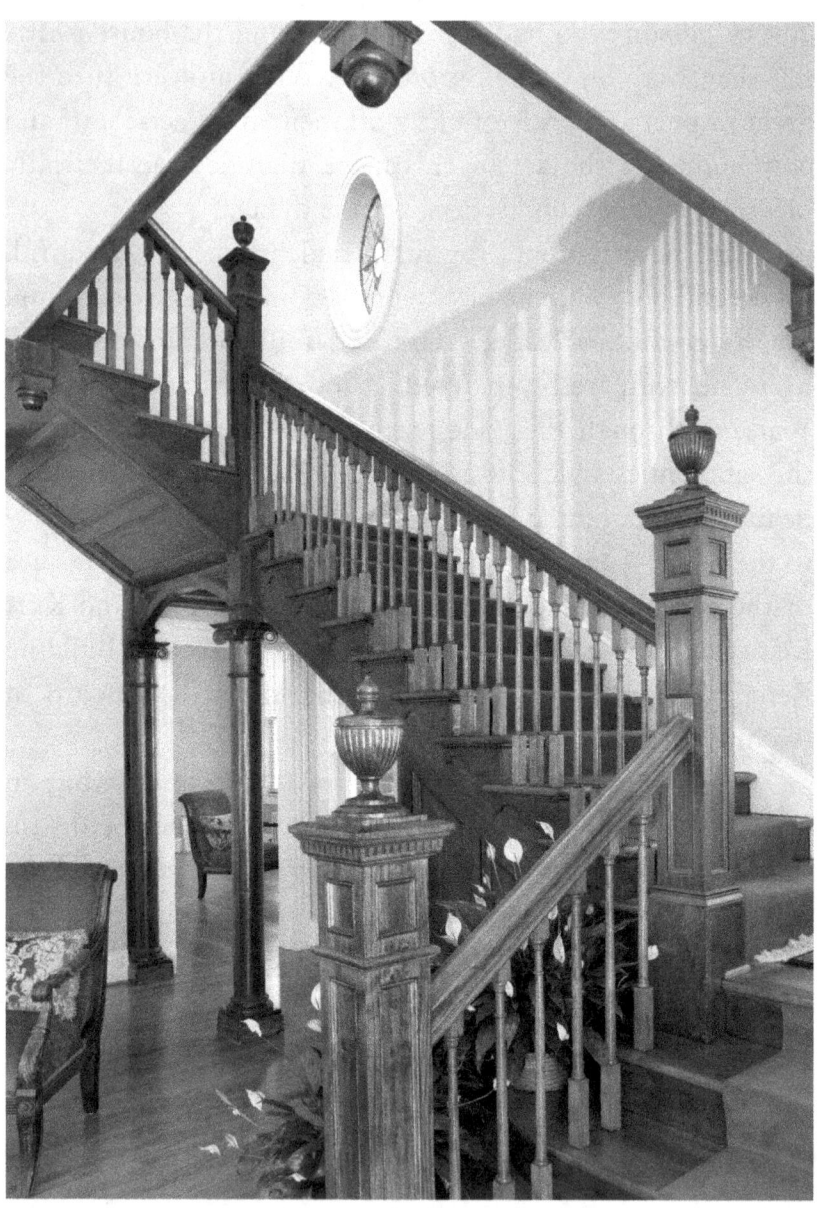

"The renovated house was beautiful, inside and out."

The early feedback from patients and their families was encouraging, but it was an August 2005 letter to Debbie Bell, RN, the Hospice House manager, that gave perhaps the most definitive answer to the question:

Dear Debbie:

You had asked my Mother to write down her thoughts about the Hospice House. She started it but never finished it … I think she didn't finish it in part because it would focus on her impending death. She didn't think about dying. She would tell her nurse, Eleanor, "Every day is a good day." 'Today' is where she spent her life, not worrying about tomorrow. Since she never finished it, and in gratitude for all you and your staff did for us, I have finished it for her …

Someone once said that in evaluating your most important relationships you should think, "Who do I want holding my hand when I die?" Sometimes that holding is symbolic and in others it is real. On July 1, 2005, at 6:07 a.m., my mother passed away peacefully at the Hospice House as my sister and I sat on either side of her holding her hands. The journey had been a gift.

At age 86 our mother was focused on life. In early spring, after a week of annoying stomach pain, she was referred to Martha Jefferson Hospital for an ultrasound. The ultrasound was followed by a cat scan. She had pancreatic cancer. A doctor we had just met sat on her bed at the hospital and told her she had three to six months to live. She laughed. "That's wonderful. I'll never get senile." The journey had begun. He mentioned chemo as an option. She dismissed the idea. "I'm fine. I've had a great life. Use your talent on the young."

We met with the Hospice liaison and discussed going home versus the Hospice House. There is something fundamental about "going home," and that was her first inclination. But, after my sister and I visited Hospice House and met Debbie, it was decided that it was the best alternative for my mother and all of us.

She walked into the house on March 23, 2005 and was led to her new room — Room 4. A beautiful room, full of sunlight from four large windows which provided a view of Park Street, the church across the way, joggers, weddings, traffic and one very special raccoon — life.

It was explained that when Hospice employees came across the threshold of her room, they were 'guests'. They weren't guests for long. All became friends. Some became family. We began to swap stories of our past and our present.

My mother was active and her pain controlled. She questioned whether she had come too early to the Hospice House. She hadn't. Being in the house gave the staff time to learn about her medically and care for her better as the disease progressed. Even more importantly, it gave time to build a relationship with her, to build her confidence to ask the questions that needed to be asked, to know her wishes would be met and to enjoy the world of being surrounded by people who genuinely care for you.

She enjoyed eating breakfast downstairs, walking the halls, going to church . . . At night when I left, she would stand at the window in her room and wave goodbye. She had always stood on the porch of her house and waved when we left. She was now doing the same thing from her new home.

As the disease progressed, she stopped coming down for breakfast and stopped going to the window. She began thanking Hospice staff with an even gentler tone. She told 'Nurse Andy', "It's about time for me to go." She slept more. My sister spent the night with her Tuesday. We both stayed Wednesday and Thursday.

In that House and room that had become her home, helped by the miracles of medicine and surrounded by her old and new family, she passed away in the way she had always hoped — loving life but not afraid of dying; teaching us how to live, not only by her life, but by her death.

The Hospice House was used as it was intended. It is not a place to go to die. It is a place with new friends waiting. Waiting to organize the unimportant things

*like medicine, food and shelter so that the resident
and family can focus on the most important things.*

*Thank you Debbie, Annie, Andy, Frank, Sue,
Loretta, Jeanie, Francis, Gay, Tammie, Eleanor,
Stephanie, Sadia and Autumn. The work you do is a
service and a gift. It helped deliver a blessed passing
to a wonderful woman and greatly touched the people
who loved her and watched your care. We will forever
be in your debt.*

At an impressive ceremony on April 17, 2009, Hospice
House was dedicated in honor of Newton and Wilma
Thomas. The couple had retired to the Charlottesville area
after many years of living and working in Colombia and
Mexico where Wilma Thomas taught elementary school and
Newton Thomas worked for and ultimately directed a major
Coca-Cola franchise. Eventually, Mr. Thomas became a
patient of Hospice of the Piedmont and, following his death,
Mrs. Thomas made a sizeable donation to the Sharing the
Journey Campaign, noting appreciation for the care received
from the hospice staff and from a very special hospice
volunteer. Combined with other gifts and generous bequests
from each of their estates, the exceptionally generous couple
contributed over $1 million to the opening and endowment
of Hospice House.

The journey to 501 Park Street had not been without bumps
and turns along the way, but with the vision, perseverance,
and generosity of a multitude of old and new friends of

Hospice of the Piedmont, the dream of an outstanding Hospice House had become a reality. Since opening its doors to receive patients on the morning of November 14, 2004, the House had quickly proved to be a wonderful addition to the community's resources for end of life care. Indeed, Debbie Bell, RN, the Hospice House manager, is accustomed to having all patient rooms occupied as well as a waiting list of patients desiring entry. Still, it was startling to hear her report that, as of September 30, 2010, a total of 305 patients had already spent the final weeks of their journey at this very special Hospice House.

Chapter 13

WATCHING LAWRENCE WELK

The capital campaign, combined with the renovation of the Park Street property and all the other work required for the opening of Hospice House in late 2004, obviously required a major commitment of time and energies from Roberta White and the members of her administrative staff. Nevertheless, significant staffing and operational changes took place during this period as well, as the search continued for more effective community outreach, and for innovative ways of meeting the needs of patients and their loved ones.

In early January 2002, Hospice of the Piedmont's in-house pharmacy became fully operational under the leadership of pharmacist Bill McCoy. Although the presence of a pharmacy is usual for hospices attached to hospitals, it is highly unusual for a freestanding, community-based hospice like Hospice of the Piedmont — another instance of innovation focused on meeting patient needs. In addition to providing Hospice with significant savings in the cost of prescription drugs, the in-house pharmacy provided patients with immediate access to hospice-related medications and, in this case, the added advantage of Bill McCoy's expertise as a compounding pharmacist. Serving as an active member of the interdisciplinary team, Bill provided significant support to the medical directors and patient physicians. He was often able to compound products that could be used in lieu of more costly traditional drugs for pain management and symptom control and, in many difficult cases, proved adept at compounding transdermal gels capable of delivering medications through the skin for very effective results.

Anne Marie Fromm, RN, an experienced and exceptional member of the nursing staff since 1993, was chosen to assume the new position of hospice nurse specialist in 2002. While retaining a caseload of patients, she would be acting as a mentor and preceptor to new staff, including physicians, nursing students and other team members. Anne's reputation for outstanding end-of-life care was well known by the staff and her elevation to the new position was applauded as well-deserved. It also served as a reminder of the high standards of care expected from each member of the clinical staff. In other staff changes that year, Chaplain Tony Perrino resigned and was replaced by David Flack.

During the spring of 2002, Jean Bradley, the director of nursing and clinical services, spent two weeks in Britain, where she attended an international study seminar on Hospice and Palliative Care in the U.K. Highlighted by a visit to St. Christopher's Hospice in London, Jean was able to see, at first hand, how hospice care had developed and grown since

Dame Cicely Saunders founded St. Christopher's in 1967. In international round table discussions and small groups, Jean discovered that "the consistent thread that binds us all together is our commitment to the dignity of each individual and the right of every person to die with minimal suffering and with the support of their loved ones."

All phases of the hospice program were growing during the years leading up to the opening of Hospice House in 2004 — *Journeys, Transitions*, social work, bereavement counseling, and the number of educational presentations given throughout the service area. The first of the *Journeys Thru the Seasons* camps was held on July 27, 2002, at the Triple C Camp, with 23 children enrolled and Chaplain Katha Bollfrasse facilitating a separate support group for parents and family members during the very meaningful event. Area schools and agencies were beginning to make referrals to the growing program, underlining the need for increased support for children who were dealing with the loss of a significant person in their lives.

It was during this time that some members of the local Senior Center volunteered to help with the *Journeys* program by making "Bearables" — small teddy bears incorporating fabric from clothing that had been worn by the child's loved one. The group of 20 ladies agreed to devote their time and skills to create these priceless treasures. Meanwhile, the 110 active Hospice volunteers were continuing to provide a cornerstone of support, working in all parts of the program. In addition to their traditional role of providing presence and practical support to hospice patients and their families and offering administrative assistance in the office, some of them were now visiting *Transitions* clients, undergoing training for serving on the Speaker's Bureau, working in the bereavement department, or receiving training from the art therapists in preparation for service as *Journeys* volunteers.

During the summer of 2003, Dean Jeanette Lancaster completed her term as president of the board and was followed in office by J. Michael Burris, the vice president and chief financial officer of Martha Jefferson Hospital. The average daily patient census, after remaining in the low 80s for some time, had begun to show a steady increase — some of it, no doubt, as a result of the unusual amount of publicity surrounding the "Sharing the Journey" campaign and a better comprehension of the services provided by Hospice of the Piedmont. By 2004, the average daily census had reached the mid 140s.

Along the way, a dramatic decrease in hospitalizations was noted. This was attributed in part to the utilization of symptom relief kits prepared by the pharmacy, and to the availability of part-time continuous care nurses. One of the strengths of Hospice of the Piedmont was its ability to hire exceptional nurses to provide continuous care when needed — a level of care in which licensed personnel attend the patient for an extended period to manage symptoms, support the family, and prevent the need for hospitalization.

The need for a larger office complex had once more become critical and, with no further space available in the Pantops building, the search began for a new location. Finding a facility with the large number of parking spaces required proved difficult, but a lease was finally negotiated for offices at 2200 Old Ivy Road, across from the Miller Center of Public Affairs. Commenting on plans for the April 2004 move, Roberta said, "Our staff is excited about the prospect of having a little more room . . . . None of us is looking forward to moving, but we hope this will be the last time for many years to come!" Upon hearing this, a 15-year staff member, for whom this would be the fourth office site since coming to Hospice of the Piedmont, shook his head and responded, "Hope springs eternal!"

Randy Rudolph, manager of human resources and jack of all trades, left Hospice at the end of May as he and his wife moved to Warrenton, Virginia. Employed initially as senior accountant, Randy had fulfilled a number of eclectic functions and, as HR manager, provided outstanding support to the staff and managers. His competency and striking wit would be greatly missed. Bob Kiefer was hired to replace him and came on board in time to receive several weeks of orientation before Randy's departure.

In a move to strengthen the grief and loss services, Tanya Givens, BSW, a bereavement social worker, was hired to be dedicated to family contact and program development for bereaved hospice family members. Plans were put in place for offering a variety of grief education presentations to the community throughout the year. Dr. Joe David, psychiatrist, agreed to participate in the projected community education series on grief and loss and to be a consultant for Hospice of the Piedmont, providing help to the counseling staff in maximizing their skills.

During the fall of 2004, chaplain staffing was increased with the addition of Pam Sivens and Sandy Sarvananda, PhD. They would be joining chaplains Katha Bollfrasse and David Flack in covering the interdisciplinary teams and co-leading a series of bereavement groups.

By the time the Hospice House opened in late 2004, Hospice of the Piedmont was experiencing a heartening upswing in several important areas. In addition to significant growth in patient census and programs, there was evidence that the arduous "Sharing the Journey" campaign had served to expand the donor base and increase awareness of the ongoing need for community support to assure the availability of this outstanding end-of-life care.

It had been a momentous year in many respects — the awarding of the Kresge challenge grant, the Hospice House construction, October's house blessing, the open house on November 7, the long-awaited opening on November 19, the Assisted Living licensure received in December, and then an outstanding Hospice Tree Celebration at First Presbyterian Church on December 12. A momentous year, indeed.

But, for all that, the age-old problem of the public image of Hospice continued to be a nagging concern. It was still common in some circles to encounter the "awkward silence" triggered by the mention of hospice. It was particularly disconcerting to encounter health care professionals and terminally ill patients who failed to understand that hospice is not about "giving up" and dying, but about living and being supported in maximizing the quality of life in the time that is left, whether it be for one week, one month, or one year.

In the continuing effort to demystify hospice, an educational brochure was produced during this period, highlighting the comments of some persons who had experienced firsthand the care provided by Hospice of the Piedmont. One of them was Barbara Price, whose mother had been a patient and, for whom she had been the caregiver.

"I found the courage to face unknown medical situations because I knew Hospice was there to help me," Barbara wrote after losing her mother. "Without the physical, emotional and spiritual support of Hospice of the Piedmont, I could not have been the caregiver I was. . . . I found the strength and stamina to care for mother at home because of the special 'angels' Hospice provided. There was the nurse who greeted my mother in the morning with a smile, the nurse's aide who bathed and massaged her, the social worker with whom I could talk, and the volunteer who offered so much support and became a family friend."

"I had trouble facing mother's death, but I also had to learn to let her live. . . . I learned that this was a time for living. Because of mother's condition, I was afraid to take her anywhere in my car. Mother loved music, particularly big band music, and I overcame my fear and took her to concerts. The last Saturday of her life, we sat together holding hands and watching Lawrence Welk on television. It's a wonderful memory and I am so grateful to Hospice of the Piedmont for helping to make it possible."

Chapter 14

NEW JOURNEYS

As Hospice of the Piedmont entered its 25th anniversary year in 2005, Roberta White was nearing the end of five extraordinary years as executive director. In her board report she reflected on all that had happened since her arrival in 2000: "I am struck by how much our organization has changed, stabilized and grown over the past five years." Then, in a prophetic assessment of what needed to happen next in the evolution of the agency, she continued, "I think this is the juncture where 'the mission' is joined by the sound business principles that assure the survival of our organization." Indeed, the next five years of her tenure would witness many internal changes in Hospice of the Piedmont as it positioned itself for a growing future.

In reporting on the activities of the *Journeys* program for children and youth and its outreach to several area schools, Roberta informed the board of a special community service Hospice of the Piedmont had provided at the Covenant School in Charlottesville. The student body had recently experienced four traumatic losses — a former student killed in Iraq, followed by the deaths of three current students in an automobile accident. At the request of school officials, Hospice of the Piedmont's *Grief and Loss* team of social workers, art therapists and volunteers provided timely on-site intervention and counseling for a number of faculty members and students as a public service.

On a personal note, Roberta paid tribute to long-time administrative assistant Judy Heyde, who had recently retired because of health problems, praising her for the invaluable services she had provided through the years. With discernible pride, Roberta saluted Assistant Director of Clinical Services Theresa O'Brien, RN, and her hard-working clinical team for the excellent reputation they had earned for timely admissions to hospice care and the extraordinary support they provided for patients and their loved ones. "The willingness and capacity of our interdisciplinary teams to be flexible in providing care to meet each family's needs, and the lengths to which they will go to accommodate those needs is a hallmark of Hospice of the Piedmont," she wrote. "This sets us apart from many other organizations that provide end-of-life care."

Highlighting the new programs and innovations that had been added during her tenure, Roberta reminded her board that "few other hospices can boast a dedicated on-call team, continuous care nurses, a hospice house, a compounding pharmacist, and support programs as comprehensive as our *Journeys*, *Transitions*, and *Grief and Loss* services."

Early in the year, Hospice of the Piedmont contracted with MCV in Richmond, offering the hospice pharmacy as an intern site. Since pharmacy schools had shifted their focus to clinical studies with very little emphasis on compounding drugs, MCV wanted a partnership where compounding was practiced. Pharmacist Bill McCoy's reputation was spreading throughout the area and he had been asked by a number of area doctors to compound transdermal medications for non-hospice patients — another instance of how the community is the winner when a hospice commits to such innovative and high-quality services.

The average daily patient census had now climbed to 150. The growth was attributed to a number of factors, including a higher visibility of the program created by the opening of Hospice House, strong working relationships with both hospitals and their physicians, and the demonstrated ability to respond to needs for hospice care in a timely fashion. Sensing that continued growth in patient census would have implications for internal structure, staffing and governance, Roberta and the board concluded that the time had come to revisit the mission, vision and values of Hospice of the Piedmont and craft a three-year strategic plan. A search was undertaken for a seasoned consultant to facilitate the process.

Following interviews with several outstanding hospice consultants, the board's executive committee recommended that the strategic planning and governance proposal of Dorothy N. Moga of Burke, Virginia, be accepted. The Board approved the recommendation and the stage was set for a three-year plan to identify key areas internally that needed to be established and/or strengthened to encourage and accommodate continued growth in the patient census.

The hospice world was saddened to learn of the death of Dame Cicely Saunders on July 14, 2005, at age 87. The remarkable founder of the modern hospice movement and pioneer in the field of palliative care died peacefully at St. Christopher's Hospice in London, the hospice she had established in 1967. As the hospice family in the Charlottesville area mourned her passing, her personal visit to Charlottesville in 1978 was remembered for providing a major impetus for the founding of Hospice of the Piedmont in 1980.

Dorothy Moga, an experienced hospice and healthcare consultant, began her work with a comprehensive assessment of all the program elements of Hospice of the Piedmont. In a meeting with the current and incoming officers of the Board, committee chairs and senior staff, she defined her role as facilitator in the planning process and set the stage for a two-day strategic planning retreat for the board and senior management in October. The purpose of the retreat was to develop ideas and establish common ground that would lead to a new statement of the mission of Hospice of the Piedmont and the formulation of a strategic plan for the way ahead.

In a presentation of current trends in nonprofit boards, Ms. Moga underlined the growing expectation that nonprofit boards have a clearer understanding of their role and responsibilities. Highlighting the trend toward smaller boards that could be more nimble in decision making and more encouraging of active participation at meetings, she proposed that the board should be driving the organization and having more substantive meetings that encouraged active discussion and debate of significant issues. Among other important trends examined was the growing number of boards with a governance committee responsible for an ongoing process of identifying the needs of the organization in its makeup — the skill sets needed, its geographic and ethnic representation, etc., and with identifying and cultivating board nominees to fill the assessed needs. She emphasized that there should be a balance between the board and CEO, as well as a mutual respect and trust in their work together. In the months ahead, the board of Hospice of the Piedmont would effectively incorporate many of these trends into its work. And so began a creative process designed to prepare and equip Hospice of the Piedmont for a growing future of service in central Virginia — a process that would involve staff, board and volunteers, with an emphasis on governance, a reassessment of staffing needs and the hiring of a chief medical officer.

The strategic planning retreat in October proved helpful in identifying areas of challenge, goals to be achieved in the future and the resources needed to succeed. It became clear that growth in the patient census was creating the need to staff at a higher level and add more administrative and clerical support throughout the organization. With that in mind, the identification of staffing needs for each department was accepted as a priority, with special attention given to areas where too much responsibility was being placed on one position. In light of the historic dependence on Medicare as a primary source of funding and the continuing pattern of decreases in Medicare reimbursement, the need for creating a fully staffed development department was seen as particularly critical. After an assessment of needs going forward, the decision was made to create the position of chief development officer to oversee all aspects of fundraising, planned giving, and donor cultivation and relationships.

During the year, notice was received from the Virginia Department of Health that new Assisted Living regulations would require the presence of an RN on each shift at Hospice House. Based on the premise that the new regulation was unnecessary in light of the present staffing of an LPN, an aide, and an on-call RN for the eight-bed facility, Hospice of the Piedmont sought, and received, a variance. However, in keeping with its mission of providing hospice care "with the highest level of skill, compassion and respect," the decision was eventually made to voluntarily provide the RN on each shift at Hospice House.

The Hospice Tree Celebration of Life was held in early December at the First Baptist Church on Park Street in Charlottesville. Using a different format, the annual memorial service, planned by Pam Sjolander, director of volunteers and bereavement, featured a series of inspiring stories narrated by hospice volunteers and staff members, followed by the lighting of the Hospice Tree and an informal reception.

2006 proved to be an extremely busy and productive year for the board and staff of Hospice of the Piedmont. During the year, Charlene Menje succeeded Faith Havran as case manager of the growing *Transitions* program for pre-hospice clients and Tina Hughey-Commers became the volunteer services coordinator. Lois Pearson joined the staff in June to serve as the executive assistant to CEO Roberta White. Over the next few years, as staffing of the various departments expanded and the role of the expanded senior leadership team became more substantive, Lois's title would transition to executive team specialist.

During the year over 700 hospice patients and their families were served and, by the time the Hospice House completed its second year of operation at the end of 2006, a total of 115 hospice patients had been cared for in that special facility. Amazingly, the clinical staff drove over 600,000 miles visiting patients in Charlottesville and the nine surrounding counties in 2006. The *Journeys* program gave comfort and support to more than 100 children and their parents who had experienced the death of a loved one and well over 1,000 families received service through one of the *Grief and Loss* programs.

Family satisfaction surveys and a gratifying stream of appreciative letters continued to underline the importance of these journey-sharing services to hospice patients and their families and the profound difference they made to human lives. Thoughtful expressions of gratitude provided the board, staff and volunteers with an encouraging validation of their work together:

"Hospice of the Piedmont transformed a time of fear, sorrow and questions into a time of warmth, peace and love for my dear wife and for me. I shall always be grateful to all of you."

"It is impossible to find words to adequately express our gratitude for everything you and your staff provided us. The scope of your program is breathtaking . . . and you were indispensable to my husband's well-being."

"You are each special, and I will be forever grateful that Hospice of the Piedmont was there to help my family through my dad's journey from this life. (He) died peacefully, and lived fully until the end. Thank you for helping him and us."

The strategic planning/governance task force had been working with the staff to evolve a cogent restatement of the mission, vision and values of Hospice of the Piedmont as it looked toward the future and positioned itself to meet the community needs for hospice services over the coming years. Out of the process, this reaffirmation of Hospice of the Piedmont's mission, vision and values, cast in simplified wording, was adopted:

MISSION

To serve our community with hospice care and supportive services related to serious illness and loss with the highest level of skill, compassion and respect.

VISION

To be the provider and the employer of choice in our community for the delivery of hospice care and supportive services related to serious illness and loss.

VALUES

We will accomplish our mission and meet the needs of the community by adhering to the following core values:

Respect
We recognize and appreciate the diversity, worth, dignity and privacy of each patient, family member, co-worker and volunteer.

Advocacy
We actively support the patient's choice for end of life care.

Integrity
We hold ourselves to the highest level of ethical conduct in every aspect of our organization.

Stewardship
We make effective and efficient use of the resources available to help us accomplish our mission.

Effectiveness
We work with individuals and organizations to ensure the most effective, compassionate, appropriate and highest quality of care available.

With the leadership of President J. Michael Burris, the fourteen-member board of directors spent many extra hours during 2006 and 2007 implementing goals of the new strategic plan being hammered out with the guidance of consultant Dorothy Moga. Much of the board's attention was focused on the question of hiring a chief medical officer and the goal of improving board governance through building a stronger, more diverse board of directors. Three new members were welcomed to the Board during this transformative time in Hospice of the Piedmont's history: Marcia Adams, Kathy Rash and John Haire. They joined continuing Board members Michael Burris, Barry Anderson, Donna Plasket, Robert Freer, Mildred Best, Maxine Burton, Pat Coffey, Elaine Kroner, Caroline McLean, Christopher McLean and Susan Mintz.

In the fall of 2006, Denise M. Kirchner, RN, MN, MPS, joined the staff as director of counseling. Denise would become a valued member of a professionally staffed senior leadership team that would be put in place over the next several years as a result of the strategic planning process.

The Hospice Tree Celebration of Life ceremony for 2006 was held at First Presbyterian Church on Park Street in early December. Following a reception afterwards, the Hospice Tree was moved across Park Street to the porch of the Hospice House, where it remained lighted until the end of the year.

At the board retreat in early January 2007, the board and members of staff heard a presentation from Martha Twaddle, MD, chief medical officer (CMO) of Midwest Palliative and Hospice Care Center in Chicago, and her CEO, Mary Sheehan, on the role of the CMO in hospice care. The retreat led to formation of a CMO task force with the goal of hiring a chief medical officer by the end of 2007. Meanwhile, board President J. Michael Burris completed his term of office during the summer of 2007 and was followed in office by Elaine Kroner.

During the year, new directors of marketing, development, and human resources were added to the senior leadership team, and a chief medical officer was appointed. Sean McCusty, with a background in the financial services industry, was named director of marketing; Karen J. Ratzlaff, an experienced coordinator of fundraising and alumni affairs efforts at the University of Virginia School of Nursing, became the director of development; Kent Hunter, a veteran human resources professional, became director of human resources; and, after serving as a medical director for three years, Dr. Timothy Short, a highly respected physician who was board certified in family medicine and palliative medicine, became Hospice of the Piedmont's first chief medical officer.

Toward year's end, two valued staff members left Hospice of the Piedmont — Sam Morgan, who had served as CFO since 2000, and Jan Phillips, director of quality. Linda Allan, MSN, a long-time staff member who had served as a field nurse and a team leader, was appointed as the new director of education and quality.

One of those remembered during the December Hospice Tree Celebration of Life at First Presbyterian Church was former hospice patient Richard "Dick" Dershimer, who had died peacefully at his home in Charlottesville on November 21, 2007. After a distinguished career in education, Dick had spent a number of years promoting hospice care, helping to establish a hospice in Syracuse, New York, helping to found a program to prepare medical professionals and lay workers to work with hospice patients, and developing workshops on grief counseling. He went on to serve as president of the New York State Hospice Association and, after moving to Charlottesville in 1989, served several terms on the board of directors of Hospice of the Piedmont, including a three-year term as president. His book *Counseling the Bereaved* (Pergamon Press, 1990) became a widely used resource in the hospice community.

2008 proved a very busy year for Hospice of the Piedmont. With the lease at 2200 Old Ivy Road in its final year, the decision on remaining there or seeking another location became a priority. Space available in the present building was no longer sufficient to house the growing staff under one roof, necessitating the rental of additional office space offsite. A systematic search was undertaken for office space that would provide a professional, secure and well-maintained environment for the expanding staff, with ample parking and easy access to the major routes used to cover the nine-county service area. The targeted search led to the signing of a five-year lease for a large suite of offices at 675 Peter Jefferson Parkway in the Pantops area. The new offices were conveniently located just off Interstate 64, and near the new Martha Jefferson Hospital then under construction and scheduled to open in the late summer of 2011. The move into the new offices was scheduled for December 2008.

Among new additions to staff during the summer was Shelley O'Connor, RN, who was named lead team leader and eventually became a member of the expanding senior leadership team. During the fall, Hospice of the Piedmont announced its sponsorship of *Piedmont Palliative Care*, a consulting service available to physicians caring for inpatients at Martha Jefferson Hospital diagnosed with challenging symptoms and illnesses but who did not yet qualify for hospice services. Consultations were also available for the care of patients at several area skilled nursing facilities — Augusta Nursing and Rehab, The Colonnades, and the Martha Jefferson Infirmary. Dr. Lisa Illig, board certified in internal medicine and hospice and palliative medicine, was named to share the palliative care responsibilities of this new service with CMO Timothy Short, MD.

In the final months of 2008, Director of Development Karen Ratzlaff initiated the quiet phase of a $3 million endowment campaign to ensure that Hospice House would remain a resource to the community for years to come. Ron Sykes, headmaster of Covenant School and the grateful son of a former Hospice House resident, agreed to lead the fundraising effort.

In accepting his leadership role in the endowment campaign, Ron said, "I think it surprises people when I say this, but I firmly believe that the last six months of Mother's life were the best of her life. She was loved, cared for, made new friends, said her goodbyes to her family — all in the nicest home she'd ever lived in. We will never be able to fully repay the gift Hospice of the Piedmont gave my mother, but we want to try."

One of the delightful events benefitting the endowment fund took place at The Greencroft Club in Ivy, Virginia, on November 12, 2008. On that evening, 65 friends and colleagues of John L. Lanham, MD, attended a surprise "roast" marking his completion of twenty years as a volunteer medical director for Hospice of the Piedmont. A highlight of the evening was the announcement that his friends and colleagues had joined members of the board and staff in contributing more than $40,000 to the "John L. Lanham Hospice House Elevator Fund." A plaque recognizing John for his faithful service "though all our ups and downs" was installed in the Hospice House elevator, and the gifts were folded into the Hospice House Endowment to ensure access to all patients in need of this facility, regardless of financial circumstances.

The early December Hospice Tree Celebration of Life and reception was held once again at First Presbyterian Church, where an overflow crowd gathered to remember and honor their loved ones and renew friendships with members of Hospice of the Piedmont's staff who had provided care for them. The eagerly anticipated move into the spacious office suite at 675 Peter Jefferson Parkway took place in mid-December, bringing the staff under one roof once more.

In February 2009, the extensive search for an outstanding chief financial officer ended with the hiring of CPA Fred Maute. An experienced businessman, Fred was coaxed out of early retirement from Music Today to assume this important post and quickly established himself as a respected member of the senior leadership team.

Through the leadership of Development Director Karen Ratzlaff, the Agnes Coburn Legacy Society was established in 2009 to honor the dedicated friends of Hospice who remembered the organization in their estate plans. The increasing emphasis on planned giving grew out of the experience of continued decreases in Medicare reimbursement and awareness that the viability of quality hospice care could not depend on the Hospice Medicare benefit for its major source of funding in the future. It was altogether fitting that "Adge" Coburn's name be attached to the society honoring those leaving a legacy to ensure the future of hospice care in central Virginia — the memorial plaque mounted in the hospice offices on East Jefferson Street following her death had said it well: "Considered the mother of Hospice of the Piedmont, 'Adge' was instrumental in its founding, generous in its support and faithful in its service as a valued member of the Board of Directors until her death in August 1991."

The spring of 2009 saw the launching of Hospice of the Piedmont's *Ambassador Program* to support the community outreach needs of the organization. A large group, including board members, staff and volunteers, agreed to be proactive in promoting awareness of hospice care in their own circles of influence, sharing accurate information, promoting Speaker's Bureau presentations, making print materials available, and the like.

Elaine Kroner completed her busy term as president of the board at the end of June and was succeeded in office by Donna Plasket. By the end of the year, the Hospice House endowment campaign had reached the halfway mark with commitments of $1.58 million. The goal for completing the $3 million campaign was set for 2011.

The year-end memorial service received a new name in 2009. The former "Hospice Tree – A Celebration of Life" was renamed "Hospice Illumination – A Community Celebration of Life" — the publicity emphasizing that the event was not solely for the hospice family, but was provided for the entire community. Once more the sanctuary of First Presbyterian Church was filled to near-capacity for the meaningful ceremony.

For some months, Director of Marketing Sean McCusty had been engaged in intensive work on the education and outreach concerns highlighted during the strategic planning process — namely, the need to work on branding issues, greater name recognition of Hospice of the Piedmont in the nine-county service area, and efforts to educate and raise community awareness of hospice care. As Roberta White phrased it, "We are dedicated to serving our whole community and want to assure that everyone who needs and wants hospice care knows who we are and what we offer."

Research in the service area revealed that, although there was a strong awareness of the presence of Hospice of the Piedmont and a very positive impression of the organization, there was also confusion about what the agency did, what services it provided, and when one should contact it for care. It was also found that many in the area would normally seek out other professionals for information related to serious illness. The research concluded that, with effective outreach to the growing elderly population in the service area, the census should move to 250 patients daily.

As a result of these findings, Sean facilitated a formal education and outreach campaign, the initial phase of which was rolled out in the early spring of 2010 in the form of a new logo and a series of professionally produced radio, TV and print media ads to be released for the 30th anniversary and to cover the entire nine-county service area.

The new logo was created in the fall of 2009 after Hospice of the Piedmont was selected to participate in the second annual Design Marathon, in which professional graphic designers, architects, and landscape architects give back to the community by providing pro-bono design services to deserving Charlottesville non-profits. With the goal of creating a new, easily recognizable image for the 30th anniversary of Hospice of the Piedmont, the design team settled on the petals of the dogwood to represent the members of the interdisciplinary teams who support patients and their families. The petals are also stylized hearts, to reflect the compassionate nature of the work.

The exceptionally well-designed ads featured various staff members and volunteers and focused on these messages:

- Hospice of the Piedmont is the organization that specializes in end-of-life care;

- The staff and volunteers of Hospice of the Piedmont are specialists with unique skills to care for and support the patients and families we serve;

- Our care goes beyond the physical needs of the patient to include the emotional, spiritual and psychological issues faced by the patient and members of the patient's family;

- Anyone can make a referral; and

- The earlier Hospice of the Piedmont is involved, the sooner its specialized care can begin supporting the unique needs of the patient and family.

Meanwhile, the patient census had grown and, by the time of the anniversary, had stabilized at a daily average of 195-200. For months, a staff committee had been planning events to celebrate the 30th anniversary of the founding of Hospice of the Piedmont in 1980. The kickoff event for the staff was a festive breakfast on the morning of January 26, 2010, followed by a number of mini-events to familiarize staff with the early beginnings of Hospice of the Piedmont and underline the reasons for proudly celebrating its thirty years of service. In the lead-up to the celebration, the anniversary committee sponsored a very well-attended Faith Community Symposium at Olivet Presbyterian Church on March 11 in support of those dealing with grief and loss issues in their faith communities.

It was a lovely spring evening in the countryside outside Charlottesville on April 23, 2010 — no doubt very much like the evening nearly 30 years before that had started it all. Only this time the setting was very different and the numbers much larger, with some 250 persons gathering at the Hilltop

Pavilion on the grounds of historic Ash Lawn-Highland for the black tie *Mountain Lights: 30th Anniversary Gala*. A festive meal was accompanied by delightful music and the announcement that a total of $118,000 had been raised for Hospice of the Piedmont.

As the dinner concluded that night, board member and acting Master of Ceremonies Glenn Rust introduced CEO Roberta White, who underlined the sharp contrast between that celebratory evening and the quiet night of May 28, 1980, when it all began — how a group of twenty persons arrived at a home outside Charlottesville that night possessed by a common dream, with no way of knowing where the dream would take them: the hard work that would be involved, the discouragements and near-failures they would encounter — or the sweet victories that would keep them going. But, determined to bring hospice care to the terminally ill and their families in Planning District 10, they chose their officers that night and named their organization *Hospice of the Piedmont.*

"On this festive occasion," she said, "it may be difficult to imagine or relate to the struggle to survive in those early years. The newsletter mailed in the summer of 1983 featured an article that began like this: 'Hospice of the Piedmont is on the brink of extinction unless financial support is forthcoming from individuals, churches, foundations and social organizations . . . . As of mid-August, we have only enough funds to operate through October.'

"So, what did they do? Well, the Board of Directors took a bold step of faith — believing that the community would support this critical service, instead of pulling back, they approved three part-time positions. They believed Hospice of the Piedmont would survive, and survive and thrive, we did.

"That same can-do spirit has played out time and again through these 30 years. In 1983, with a skeleton staff and a few volunteers, they cared for a total of 55 patients and their families. Today, with a staff of 150 specialists and 160 trained volunteers, we are caring for more than 1,000 patients and their families each year, with a daily census of nearly 200 patients in our hospice program alone.

"Through thick and thin, the spirit and passion of those visionaries in 1980 lives on. It has been present in so many ways — when we expanded our service area beyond Region 10 to the nine counties we now cover; when we became a Medicare-certified hospice provider in 1988; when we became one of the few hospices in America to operate our own pharmacy; when we committed ourselves to provide support for area children and adolescents in their journey through grief and loss of a loved one.

"It was there when we mounted a multi-million dollar campaign to open the area's first Hospice House for residential care that today provides a model for others to follow; and when we expanded staff and resources to provide bereavement services throughout our service area that now support more than 1,200 clients each year, whether or not their loved one died in hospice care; and when we added a *Transitions* program for pre-hospice clients that currently

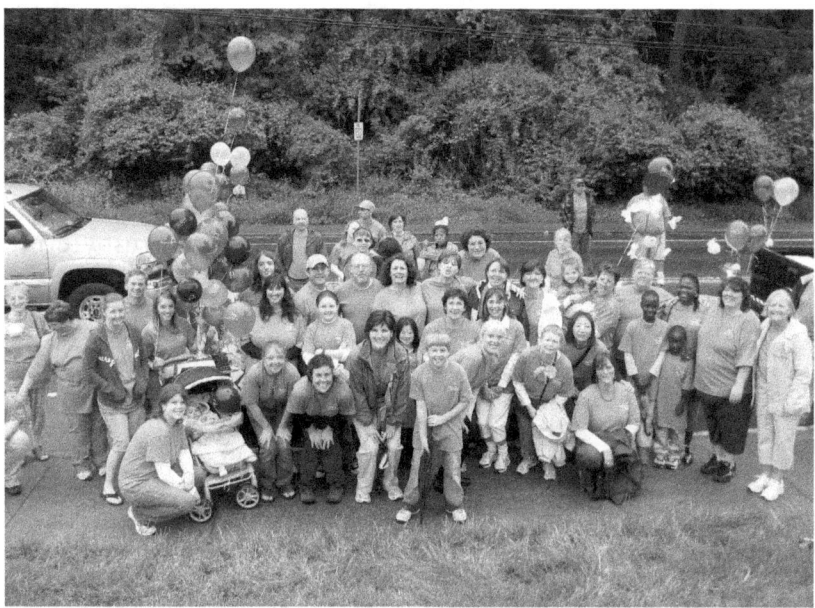

Hospice family gathered for the 2010 Dogwood Parade.

helps a daily average of 140 persons remain independent and in their homes; and when we hired our first chief medical officer and took the plunge to offer *Piedmont Palliative Care* consultations for the area.

"As I stand at the helm of this incredible organization today, I could not be more proud of the dedication and pride shown by our staff, volunteers and board of directors as they work to ensure that all that was envisioned 30 years ago, and all that has been created in the intervening years, is secure and available to anyone in need, and that it remains centered on our mission to serve this community with skill, compassion and respect.

"With the continued support of caring people like you in our community, I have no doubt that the same kind of can-do spirit that has marked our past will be there for the next 30 years!"

The busy day that followed the gala began with an early morning Kiwanis Pancake Breakfast at First Presbyterian Church benefiting Hospice of the Piedmont's *Journeys* program, followed by a first-ever participation in the annual Dogwood Festival Parade in downtown Charlottesville. A remarkable number of staff, volunteers, spouses and children, and a smattering of family dogs, walked or rode in the parade, many of the adults wearing the new, brightly colored Hospice of the Piedmont shirts and carrying signs highlighting its many services. The long day continued with attendance at the Foxfield Spring Race Meet, where Hospice of the Piedmont was a welcome beneficiary.

Yet to come was participation by staff members and volunteers in the Scottsville Independence Parade in July and Alzheimer's Memorial Walks in Charlottesville and Staunton in the fall of 2010. But the event that seemed to put a "period" and an "exclamation point" on the 30th anniversary celebrations for the staff, board, and volunteers was the picnic out in the countryside on Saturday afternoon, September 18th. Amid the laughter, camaraderie, and replaying of the events of the year, one could sense a readiness to move on.

On Monday morning, members of the staff arrived for work and walked past the front desk as receptionist Sonya

Hamilton was dealing with a rush of incoming calls, just as she had done each workday morning for nearly ten years:

"Hospice of the Piedmont — how may we help you?"

They headed down the hallway, taking the first steps toward the next 30 years and new journeys to be shared.

REMEMBERING
TO REMEMBER

In the old Victorian house on East Jefferson Street, one needed neither clock nor calendar to know that the week was about to end. The noise downstairs announced it, loud and clear — a growing cacophony as, one after another, the field staff returned from patient visits and gathered in the small kitchen. Peals of laughter swept down the hallway and up the stairwell to my second-floor office. No doubt about it — it was Friday, the end of another week.

At first, I mildly resented the weekly intrusion of noise but, as time went on, found myself actually looking forward to it. Glancing up from my computer monitor, I would smile to myself as the weekly ritual got underway. Goodness knows, all of them had dealt with enough during the week to justify the need for laughter and the corny jokes they loved to tell. Enough human sorrow and enough tears, enough physical needs to be tended and spiritual quests to be honored, enough fears to be assuaged and regrets to be heard, enough affirmations of faith for what lay ahead, interspersed with some precious moments when the grandeur of the human spirit brightened the room, and the only fitting response was the gift of one's presence. All this, and more, they brought to the Friday gathering.

It seemed a weekly catharsis of sorts, an emptying, a commitment of the events of the past week — and a kind of victory celebration that they had been able to do what was needed, had done it to the best of their abilities, and had come through it all intact. In some profound sense, it was a weekly reminder of who we were, what we were about, and what, at best, hospice care was meant to be — a true sharing of the journey. After the staff had returned to their cars and headed home for the weekend, a strange kind of joy lingered in the air.

That seems long ago — we're a much larger family now, with a staff of 150 — and Friday afternoon sounds don't carry here nearly so well as they did in the old house. We've grown so large, so much has changed and we are busy trying to keep up with it all. But one thing has not changed over these past thirty years — to be invited to share one of life's most important journeys with others is still a very high privilege. In the midst of all the other changes, that remains constant.

Sure, Friday afternoons are different now — the family has outgrown the kitchen! But the need to remember who we are as a hospice family, what we are about, and the tremendous difference it makes to human lives — this is something we will never outgrow.

EARLIEST LIST OF OFFICERS AND BOARD MEMBERS

Board Members

Dr. Martin Albert .... Physician

Mrs. Imogene Bunn... RN (retired)

Rev. C. W. Carnan .... Episcopal Priest

Mrs. Alvin F. Coburn........................... Housewife and RN

Dr. George Cooper.. Physician

John Stewart Darrell .... Investment Counselor

Carr Dorman .... Banker

Miss Betty Jo Elliott.. RN

Dr. H. Cowen Ellis.................................... Baptist Minister

Father William Gardner .... R.C. Priest

Dr. Charles Gleason .... Physician

Mrs. Asha Greer .... Nursing Student

John Groome .... Funeral Director

Father Thomas Hart .... R.C. Priest

Mrs. Rosemary Hayes... RN

Mrs. Sarah Hendley .... Social Worker

Peyton Humphrey .... Lawyer and Accountant

Dr. James G. Knight.. Physician

Mrs. Byrd Leavell.. Housewife
Mrs. Pat Llewellyn .... R.C. Eucharistic Min
Reginald Marshall .... H.E.W. Retiree
Mrs. Mary McGee............................... Public Health Nurse
John Metz.. Pharmacist
Thomas J. Michie, Jr. .... Lawyer and State Senator
Dr. William Sandusky .... Physician
Mrs. Nancy Stamm... Lawyer
William T. Stevens .... Realtor
Mrs. Robert Stewart .... Social Worker
Miss Agatha Van de Erve......................... RN Radiotherapy
Dr. Clyde Watson.. Physician
Mrs. Viola Wingfield.............................. Admin. Educator
Paul Wood .... Funeral Director
Dr. Chris Zazakos, Jr. .... Oncologist (first Medical Director)

Officers
Chairman... Dr. George Cooper
Vice-Chairman... Mrs. Asha Greer
Secretary .... Mrs. Alvin Coburn
Treasurer... John Stewart Darrell

*Concerning the use in these lists of titles such as "Miss" and "Mrs.",
since we would not have been able to find a correct alternative name
or form of address in every case, we have given the names exactly as
set down in the original records.

BOARD PRESIDENTS, 1980–2010

Dr. George Cooper 1980–1983

Dr. William R. Sandusky 1983–1985

Edmund W. Morris 1985–1986

John R. Metz 1986–1988

Mrs. Susan Garrett 1988–1990

Gerald V. "Jerry" Bailey 1990–1992

Richard A. Dershimer 1992–1995

John F. Harlan, Jr. 1995–1997

Bruce B. Galloway 1997–1999

Mrs. Frances Bonardi 1999–2002

Dean Jeanette Lancaster 2002–2004

J. Michael Burris 2004–2007

Mrs. Elaine Kroner 2007–2009

Mrs. Donna Plasket 2009–

Appendix C
THE FIRST VOLUNTEER TRAINING GROUPS

Sarah P. Hendley moved to Charlottesville in 1979, shortly after receiving her masters in social work from Catholic University in Washington, D.C. She attended Hospice of the Piedmont's first volunteer training group in 1980, was an early board member and, among many other tasks, served as volunteer coordinator until 1982. Through the years, she had saved the old Charlottesville telephone directory, in the back of which she had carefully recorded the names of those attending the first three volunteer training groups. She was kind enough to share this treasure for use in *Sharing the Journey*:

The first hospice volunteer training group was held April–June 1980. I attended it as well as Pam Fox, Jean Harvey, June Kerr, Mary Kirwin, Scott Krebs, Kate LaRue, Barbara McLaughlin, Mary Murray, Pat Llewellyn, Barbara Rich, Emma Jean Synder, and Ruth Synder.

The second hospice volunteer training group was held from January to April 1981. Mambers of the group were Joan Barnochy, Debbie Blackwell, Buck Carnan, Robia

Collins, Lenette Crescimanno, Margaret Good, Mary Harison, Sarah Gilbert, Mary Hynes, Zita Kelly, Judy Mandell, Bill Percy, Hilda Porter, Margaret Robinson, Joel Silverman, Camille Sweeney, Jo Gail Wenzel, Carol Wiegers, and Eileen Wilkins.

The third volunteer training program was held September–December 1981. The participants were Faith Argaud, Karen Collins, Ned Evans, Colleen Fitzpatrick, Beverly Gibson, John Groome, Sandra Kulund, Nancy Leavell, Dona Lewin, Altha Parr, John Parr, Mary Agnes Rhinelander, Diana Saunders, Terry Saunders, Michael Schwartz, and John Walsh.

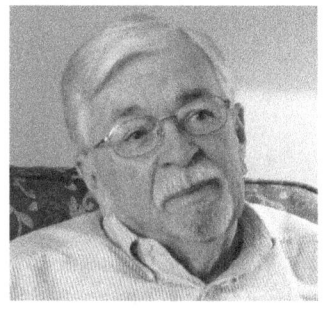

About the Author

ROBERT TALMADGE HAYNES — affectionately known as "Tal" — came to Hospice of the Piedmont in the summer of 1989, after taking early retirement from a pastoral ministry to do some writing. Shortly after his retirement, Tal had lunch with a friend who asked if he could do some part-time work for the Hospice of the Piedmont. That part-time effort, expected to last twelve weeks, concluded 21½ years later.

Tal soon became Hospice of the Piedmont's Director of Development, a title that eventually was changed to Director of Community Relations. He is most proud of his work in helping Hospice of the Piedmont realize its dream of creating a Hospice House. Tal successfully led the first major capital campaign for Hospice House at a time when the nation and the economy were reeling from the September 11th attacks. During his tenure, Tal was also responsible for starting the *Dining Around the Area* fundraiser, and the Hospice Tree of Lights. Numerous other development and marketing initiatives still bear his mark and attest to his skill with language and his drive to sustain the organization and its mission. Tal's final endeavor for Hospice brought him back to the passion that had prompted his first retirement — the love of writing. He has channeled that passion into this book documenting Hospice of the Piedmont's first 30 years.

According to Tal, "The most satisfying work a person can do is work that has a lasting impression on human life." In recognition of his invaluable contributions to the organization, in 2011 Hospice of the Piedmont dedicated one of its Quiet Rooms, set aside for counseling and consultations, to Tal.

"During the writing of the book," Tal says, "I was greatly appreciative of the patience of my wife, Barbara, and grateful for the calming presence of Amanda and Gavin, our retired racing greyhounds."